HAS SEX EDUCATION FAILED OUR TEENAGERS?

A Research Report

HAS SEX EDUCATION FAILED OUR TEENAGERS?

A Research Report

by Dinah Richard, Ph.D.

Focus on the Family Publishing
Pomona, CA 91799

First Printing, 1990
Printed in the United States of America

Dinah Richard
Has Sex Education Failed Our Teenagers?
A Research Report

Summary: A study of the effects of sex education on the rates of teenage pregnancy, sexually transmitted diseases, and abortions.

ISBN 0-929608-22-4

Focus on the Family Publishing
Rolf Zettersten, Vice President
Dean Merrill, Vice President, Communications
Wes Haystead, Curriculum Editor

TEST YOUR KNOWLEDGE ABOUT SEX EDUCATION

1. From 1971 to 1981, how much federal money was spent on family planning?
Answer: Over $2 billion. (See page 4.)

2. How successful was this investment in reducing teen pregnancies and teen abortions?
Answer: Not successful—there was a 48.3% increase in teen pregnancies and a 133% increase in teen abortions. (See page 5.)

3. How aware are advocates of adolescent family planning that their own programs contribute to promiscuity?
Answer: Very aware—here are just a few prominent people who have stated that family planning is correlated to promiscuity:

   - **Dr. Alan Guttmacher, former president of Planned Parenthood;**

   - **Dr. Robert Kistner of Harvard University (developer of "the Pill");**

   - **Dr. Kingsley Davis of Zero Population Growth;**

   - **Dr. Min Chueh Chang (one of the inventors of "the Pill");**

   - **Randomly selected physicians and psychiatrists;**

   - **The National Research Council. (See pages 11, 12.)**

4. Does the discussion of contraceptives in a classroom setting contribute to promiscuity?
Answer: Yes, according to several studies. (See pages 21, 22.)

5. Does regular use of "the Pill" solve the teen pregnancy problem?
Answer: No. The failure rate for teens who regularly use "the Pill" is much higher than for older women who regularly use it. Some studies report the failure rate for teens to be as high as 18%. (See pages 23, 24.)

6. Should teens be taught about condoms and "safe sex" in order to prevent the spread of AIDS?
Answer: Condom usage will not prevent the spread of AIDS. One study showed that the condom failure rate for preventing the transmission of AIDS was as high as 17% in a relatively short time span. (See pages 24-26.)

7. Is sex education harmful to elementary-aged children?
Answer: Yes. Child development experts confirm that explicit sex education should not be taught during the latency period. (See pages 28, 29.)

8. How capable are teenagers of making and acting upon logical decisions regarding sexual conduct?

Answer: Not very. Adolescents are still in the concrete state of cognitive development, not yet in the formal operations stage. Thus, they do not yet make decisions on a strictly rational basis. (See pages 31-33.)

9. Are most teenagers sexually active?

Answer: No. Numerous studies have shown that half of all teens graduating from high school are still virgins. Also, a high number of teens who have experienced intercourse return to abstinence. (See page 42.)

10. Which states require the teaching of abstinence education?

Answer: In 1988, California, Washington, Illinois, and Indiana passed laws requiring it. (See page 45.)

11. Is abstinence education the same as teaching religion?

Answer: No. The Supreme Court ruled in 1988 that federal funding of abstinence education for public schools does not violate the Establishment Clause. The Court declared that the teaching of abstinence is not inherently religious. (See page 47.)

12. Is abstinence education effective in inner-city schools?

Answer: Yes. Effective programs have been developed which aid teens at high risk. (See page 48.)

13. Should both abstinence and contraceptive education be provided to give a balanced approach?

Answer: No. The inclusion of information on contraceptive usage weakens the impact of abstinence education, encouraging young people to continue or begin sexual activity. (See pages 52, 53.)

14. Does abstinence education actually change the attitudes of adolescents and help to reduce the teenage pregnancy problem?

Answer: Yes. The U.S. Department of Health and Human Services has funded and tested programs across the country which prove the effectiveness of abstinence education. (See pages 56-61.)

15. Are parents willing and able to get involved in the process of educating their children about sex when abstinence is recommended?

Answer: Yes. Abstinence education has tangible and effective means of involving parents. (See pages 65-67.)

16. Does parental involvement in sex education help in reducing adolescent pregnancy?

Answer: Yes. (See pages 68-72.)

17. What about AIDS education—are there appropriate classroom resources which are based on the abstinence perspective?

Answer: Yes. (See page 92.)

SUMMARY

The teenage sexuality crisis in the United States has been characterized by a phenomenal increase in pregnancies, abortions, illegitimate births, sexually transmitted diseases, and psychological problems associated with sexual activity. Decision makers have explored various intervention programs for teens at high risk, and they have met with varying degrees of success.

The most common approach to the adolescent pregnancy problem has been family planning services available through community clinics. Under the assumption that the services would resolve the problem, the federal government allocated large amounts of money for such programs. Though the intent of the program was to help reduce the problem, that has not occurred.

Both at federal and state levels, increased funding of family planning has been correlated with an increase in teen sexual activity, pregnancies, and abortions. Though the birth rate has declined in certain locations, it is often due to a reliance on abortion rather than contraception.

The failure of adolescent family planning services is often attributed to teens' lack of accessibility to the services. However, the claim seems unfounded in view of the statistics showing that teens are using family planning services in record numbers, yet the rate of pregnancies and abortions still rises.

The failure of adolescent family planning services is also attributed to the sporadic use of contraceptives. Though irregular usage will play a role in the pregnancy outcome, consistent usage of contraceptives does not ensure pregnancy prevention. Several studies show that teens who regularly use oral contraceptives have a failure rate that is four to five times greater than the failure rate for older women.

Besides family planning services to teens, other intervention programs have been attempted. More recently, school-based clinics have been introduced onto campuses, but they have met with the same failure as family planning services elsewhere in the community.

Comprehensive sex education, particularly in the form of "values-neutral" decision making, has been adopted into the classroom. Not only has this not reduced the problem of teenage pregnancy, it has been positively correlated to an increase in adolescent sexual activity, abortion, sexually transmitted diseases, and accompanying psychological problems.

Now is the time for professionals in the field of education and health to consider innovative programs that depart from the unsuccessful attempts of the past. When designing new intervention programs, much greater success is being achieved when accurate theories of adolescent cognitive and moral development are used as the basis. A directive approach is successful because it clearly moves teens toward responsible conduct and good health. An approach which teaches refusal skills is successful because it equips teens with techniques which can be applied to realistic situations. A morally based approach is successful because it helps teens discover that all decisions have ethical considerations.

Abstinence education is based on these successful approaches. In 1981, Congress passed the Adolescent Family Life Act in order to help launch abstinence education across the country. Grants were given to help underwrite pilot programs which promote parental involvement in the educational process and teach the benefits of sexual restraint to adolescents.

Many people have wondered whether abstinence can be taught in the public school since it coincides with the values taught by the major religions. That question was resolved in 1988 when the Supreme Court ruled that abstinence education was *not* inherently religious in nature, and therefore it **could** be taught in public institutions as a major means to address the adolescent pregnancy crisis.

California, Washington, Illinois, and Indiana have passed laws requiring sex education to be taught from an abstinence perspective. Other states are currently considering the adoption of similar legislation.

Abstinence education has been shown to have a positive impact on teens' attitudes toward chastity and on their abilities to say "no" to sexual activity. Moreover, it has effectively reduced the teenage pregnancy rate in many communities.

Parental involvement is vital in helping to reduce the teenage sexuality crisis. Many abstinence programs have developed tangible and effective means of drawing parents into the process of educating their children.

Not only is abstinence education effective, it has been well received by educators, students, and parents. Commercially prepared abstinence resources such as curricula, audiovisual aids, books, and pamphlets are readily available for public school usage.

THE AUTHOR

Dinah Richard holds a Ph.D. in speech communication from Louisiana State University. She taught as a graduate assistant at L.S.U., then as a lecturer at the University of Texas at San Antonio. She and her husband, Conrad, have four children and reside in San Antonio.

For several years she directed a speaker's bureau, providing public schools and other groups with programs about the values of sexual abstinence for teenagers and the consequences of premarital sex. In response to a growing number of inquiries from teachers, counselors, and school health officials, Dr. Richard began intensive research into the comparative effectiveness of abstinence education and the contraceptive approach.

PREFACE:
THE TEENAGE SEXUALITY CRISIS

According to Planned Parenthood, **over 1 million teenage girls become pregnant each year in the United States, the highest rate in the Western world.** Other adolescent sexual issues have also come to the forefront in recent years, including an epidemic of sexually transmitted diseases (STDs), education to prevent the spread of AIDS, the establishment of school-based clinics, and the advertising of contraceptives.

In response to these problems, national and state government agencies, school officials, and community social service organizations have conducted research and developed projects targeted at adolescents and their high-risk behaviors. Often, decision makers are bombarded with so many proposals from seemingly credible sources that they are unable to analyze them all carefully. Thus, resources that consolidate the information and give guidance based on statistical findings can be of great benefit.

The purpose of this report is to provide to school personnel, community leaders, parents, medical workers, policy makers, and other interested people the information they need to assess the successes and failures of past programs dealing with the teenage sexuality crisis. It is also meant to help them realize the need to adopt innovative and successful programs. The report contains a history of past programs, summaries of major studies in the area of adolescent sexuality, evidence to support the value of enlightened approaches, and extensive lists of resources for classroom usage. Finally, the report is intended to encourage us all to work together in helping today's youth improve their lives.

CONTENTS

ACKNOWLEDGMENTS

Any work such as this has to be a team effort, and I am deeply grateful to the many people whose support helped make this report possible. I want to thank these experts who read through the manuscript and suggested improvements and corrections:

- Reed Bell, M.D., Gulf Breeze, Florida
- Nabers Cabaniss, Washington D.C.
- J. Thomas Fitch, M.D., and Laurie Fitch, San Antonio, Texas
- Lewis Hicks, M.D., Lexington, Kentucky
- David Larson, M.D., M.S.P.H., Duke University Medical Center
- Joe McIlhaney, M.D., Austin, Texas
- Barrett Mosbacker, Headmaster, Covenant Day School, Matthews, North Carolina
- Anne Newman, San Antonio, Texas
- S. DuBose Ravenel, M.D., High Point Infant & Child Clinic, Inc., High Point, North Carolina

The following individuals and organizations graciously allowed me to reprint their charts: American Life League, *The Education Reporter*, Wanda Franz, Josh McDowell Ministries, Dr. Terrance Olson, Project Respect.

I thank the following individuals and organizations which allowed me to extensively cite their research: Dr. Jacqueline Kasun, Josh McDowell Ministries, Barrett Mosbacker, Dr. Terrance Olson.

The following individuals and organizations shared helpful information which was used in this report: Citizens for Excellence in Education, Concerned Women for America, Couple to Couple League, J. Thomas Fitch, M.D., Family Research Council, Fertility Appreciation for Families, Josh McDowell Ministries, Louise Kaegi, Tom Landiss, Martha Long, Dr. Onalee McGraw, Cathy Mickels, Eric Miller, Linda Moore, Anne Newman, Terrance Olson, Project Respect, Dr. DuBose Ravenel, Respect, Inc., Teen-Aid, Womanity, and Marjorie Zimmerman.

Next, I thank the special people at Focus on the Family who were so helpful: Linda Gurrola, Wes Haystead, Janet Kobobel, Angela Najera, Diane Passno, Bruce Peppin, and Larry Weeden.

Dr. Tom Fitch and his wife, Laurie, stood beside me throughout this project and put me in touch with the people I needed to talk to. Their assistance was invaluable.

Finally, I gratefully acknowledge my husband, Conrad, my helpmate and motivator. If not for his loving support, I never would have attempted this work.

I. *FAMILY PLANNING PROGRAMS FOR ADOLESCENTS*

During the past two decades, family planning has become a common social service available through government and private health care agencies. Originally designed to help married couples determine the size of their families and spacing of children, family planning has been extended to unmarried teenagers who wish to engage in sexual activity without the consequences of pregnancy or disease.

Because teenage pregnancy was rampant, and convinced that their solution would help in the crisis, proponents of family planning carried their philosophy and programs into major institutions across the country, including the schools. Few people realize the tremendous influence family planners have had in shaping the views of policy makers, and even fewer have questioned either the appropriateness or effectiveness of contraceptive programs for teens. Yet, when decision makers analyze the history, cost, accessibility, and ineffectiveness of family planning for unmarried adolescents, they will discover the need to consider options other than family planning, school-based clinics, and contraceptive sex education.

A. HISTORY OF FAMILY PLANNING IN CONTEMPORARY AMERICA

In the post-World War II years, when servicemen returned home, married, and started families, the "baby boom" signified an unprecedented population growth in the United States. Beginning in the late 1940s and ending in the early 1960s, the boom brought about a major emphasis on families and children and was considered an asset to the American lifestyle.

By the early 1960s, the population growth in America had tapered off. In spite of that, some people expressed continuing alarm about the notion of the "population bomb." To combat the potential population explosion, groups began to petition Congress to take action. In the mid 1960s, as part of the "War on Poverty," the Office of Economic Opportunity gave family planning grants to community action agencies.[1] Surprisingly, nobody questioned why the funding was given at a time when the birthrate for all groups of American women, including teenagers, had declined.[2] Yet, the funding did not stop there. In 1967, Congress amended the Social Security Act to provide funds for family planning in maternal and child care programs, and in 1970, Congress passed the Family Planning Services and Population Research Act, amending Title X of the Public Health Services Act to make it the largest ongoing federal source of funds for contraceptives. The uniqueness of the 1970 legislation was that it included funding of contraceptives for sexually active unmarried minors.[3]

The belief that teenage pregnancy was a major social problem prompted President Richard Nixon's Commission on Population Growth and the American Future to sponsor special *Research Reports*. In 1972, the first edition made it clear that the population could be reduced by **eliminating births to unmarried teens,** and it recommended **birth control information and services and comprehensive sex education for teens.** It also advocated **voluntary sterilization and abortions on request at public expense.**[4] A year later, in 1973, abortion on demand became possible through the Supreme Court decision in Roe v. Wade.

Helping to bring about these revolutionary changes, Planned Parenthood Federation of America developed a five-year plan for the years 1976-80, stating that its mission was "to serve as the nation's foremost agent of social change in the area of reproductive health and well being." It sought to remove legal, regulatory, and cultural restrictions to "universal reproductive freedom," labeling any obstructions as "arbitrary and outmoded restrictions." Planned Parenthood also launched a major public awareness thrust to promote its philosophy.[5]

The first major step in Planned Parenthood's media campaign came in 1976, when its research arm, the Alan Guttmacher Institute, published *11 Million Teenagers: What Can Be Done About the Epidemic of Adolescent Pregnancies in the United States.*[6] The pamphlet, widely distributed at government expense, helped to promote Planned Parenthood's philosophy and programs. Frederick Jaffe, late president of the Guttmacher Institute, assured public officials that if Planned Parenthood and other family planning agencies were provided with increased federal funding, they could reduce the teenage pregnancy problem.[7]

To push the issue further, in 1977, Planned Parenthood, Zero Population Growth, and other groups published *Planned Births, the Future of the Family and the Quality of Life: Towards a Comprehensive National Policy and Program.* Designed to promote a reduction in teen pregnancies and births, the groups called for:

1. a national network for early pregnancy detection;

2. school-based education programs;

3. community information and outreach programs; and

4. programs to encourage hospitals to provide abortions.

Moreover, they demanded that Congress **provide $800 million annually by 1981.**[8]

Nobody challenged these groups, nor did Congress seem aware that though the teenage pregnancy rate hadn't decreased, the **teen birth rate had declined rapidly during this time.** Nevertheless, Congress increased funding for existing programs as well as approved the Adolescent Pregnancy Act of 1978.[9]

By this point, a decade of federal funding of family planning had passed, yet the problem of adolescent pregnancy hadn't disappeared. In 1981, the Guttmacher Institute issued another alarming publication, *Teenage Pregnancy: The Problem That Hasn't Gone Away,* calling for an even greater extension of the same programs.[10] But for the first time, opposing views were appearing at key places within the federal government. In 1981, newly elected President Reagan appointed conservative officials to serve in his cabinet and within the various executive departments. The same year, Congress passed the Adolescent Family Life Act, which helped to set a new direction in tackling the adolescent pregnancy problem. Rather than having as a primary emphasis the promotion of contraceptives for teens, this law, administered by the Office of Adolescent Pregnancy Programs, stressed that grants would be given to agencies that promoted abstinence and parental involvement.[11]

Family planning groups were not deterred during the Reagan administration. In 1985, when federal family planning appropriations were up for consideration, the Guttmacher Institute published its strongest crisis report yet. In *Teenage Pregnancy in Developed Countries: Determinants and Policy Implications,* it analyzed the issue in thirty-seven developed countries and closely compared the United States to five other Western nations. Concluding that the United States had the highest teenage pregnancy rate, the Institute blamed the American problem on:

1. irregular and inexpert use of contraceptives by American teens;

2. weak sex education programs;

3. lack of national health services; and

4. reactions of conservative religious groups.[12]

The media quickly picked up on the issue. Major news magazines and television networks ran feature stories about "kids having kids" and "children having children."[13] And with the epidemic spread of STDs among teenagers and the fear of AIDS, people began to hear about "safe sex."

As the notion of safe sex became popular in the late 1980s, major medical associations joined in campaigns to address the teen sexuality crisis. For example, the American College of Obstetricians and Gynecologists put out a pamphlet endorsing oral contraceptives for sexually active teens. It also sponsored television commercials with the same message.[14] The American Academy of Pediatrics supported similar measures and endorsed school-based clinics in areas where adequate health care is not already available.[15]

Boosting the view that family planning was favored by most professional organizations, the National Research Council published the 1987 report *Risking the Future: Adolescent Sexuality, Pregnancy and Childbearing*. Not surprisingly, the report advocated contraceptive services for teens at low or no cost, unrestricted abortion and contraceptives for teens without parental consent, condom distribution programs, and school-based clinics. This was done despite its pointing out a correlation between increased rates of sexual activity and provision of family planning to adolescents, along with an acknowledgment that this may be a causal relationship.[16]

As the United States enters the 1990s, if these trends continue, additional reports will no doubt be released, and further legislation will be introduced calling for even stronger measures. And by reading the publications, hearing the major proposals, and seeing the legislation being advocated by credible national organizations, decision makers might be led to believe that adolescent family planning services are needed now more than ever and that the government needs to extend its funding of such programs. But before drawing what seems to be a logical conclusion, policy makers need to ask how much has already been poured into family planning for teens and to what effect.

Table 1
Significant Events in the History of Contemporary Family Planning

Year	Event	Significance
1945-60	Post-World War II baby boom	Unprecedented population growth in U.S.
Early 1960s	End of baby boom	Decline in population for all categories of women in the U.S.
mid 1960s	"Population bomb" scare Office of Economic Opportunity gives family planning grants to community action agencies	Fear of overpopulation in the U.S. Beginning of federal funding of family planning groups
1967	Congress amends Social Security Act	More federal funding for family planning by way of maternal and child health programs
1969	President Nixon appoints Commission on Population Growth and the American Future	Special interest groups given the opportunity to serve on government commissions
1970	Congress passes Family Planning Services and Population Research Act, Amending Title X of the Public Health Services Act	The largest source of federal funding for family planning: for the first time, includes contraceptives for teens

1972	Commission on Population Growth and the American Future releases its first *Research Reports*	Emphasis on reducing teen births through contraceptives, abortion, sterilization, and sex education
1973	Roe v. Wade case goes before the Supreme Court	Court rules that women have a right to abortion-on-demand
1976	Planned Parenthood releases its 5-year plan	Major thrust to promote universal reproductive freedom and to introduce teens to contraceptives, abortion, sterilization, and sex education
1977	Guttmacher Institute publishes *11 Million Teenagers*	Effective publication promoting the need for Planned Parenthood's programs
1977	Planned Parenthood et. al, releases *Planned Births*	Demands Congress provide $800 million annually for family planning in the U.S.
1978	Congress increases funding for existing family planning programs and passes the Adolescent Pregnancy Act of 1978	More federal funding to family planning agencies such as Planned Parenthood
1981	Guttmacher Institute publishes *Teenage Pregnancy: The Problem*...	Further pleas for federal funding
1981	Congress passes the Adolescent Family Life Act, which is administered through the Office of Adolescent Pregnancy Programs	Emphasis on abstinence education and parental involvement to reduce teen pregnancies
1985	Guttmacher Institute publishes *Teenage Pregnancy in Developed Countries*	Foremost publication and media blitz to push for contraceptive programs and progressive sex education for teens; attack on religious fundamentalists who oppose their views
late 1980s	ACOG, AAP, and other major medical associations speak up	Call for contraceptive approach to reduce the teenage pregnancy problem
1987	National Research Council publishes *Risking the Future*	Calls for greater efforts at promoting contraceptives for teens

B. THE COST OF FAMILY PLANNING PROGRAMS FOR ADOLESCENTS

Over the past two decades, family planning groups have lobbied for and received extensive federal funding for contraceptive programs for teens. As early as 1968, $13.5 million had been allocated for family planning. Ten years later, in 1978, that amount had risen to $279 million,[17] representing a twenty-fold increase. From 1971 to 1981, total federal expenditures on family planning (exclusive of state and local funding) **exceeded $2 billion dollars,**[18] **representing an increase of 306 percent.**[19] In 1985 alone, the federal government spent over $622 million on family planning programs.[20] Table 2 shows the extensive list of federal programs as of 1986 and their sizable yearly budget.[21]

Table 2
Federal Programs Through the U.S. Department of HHS
That Address the Problem of Adolescent Pregnancy (1986)

Program	Service	Cost
Adolescent Family Life Demonstration Program through Title XX of the Public Health Service Act	Supports research and innovative, family-centered approaches to prevent teen sexual activity, reduce adolescent pregnancy, and develop effective approaches for delivering comprehensive services for pregnant adolescents and adolescent parents.	$15 million FY 1986
Family Planning under Title X of the Public Health Service Act	Provides individuals of reproductive age, including adolescents, with free or inexpensive contraceptives, infertility services, and general reproductive health care through more than 4,000 clinics around the country.	$147 million FY 1986
Maternal and Child Health Block Grant through Title V of the Social Security Act	Funds prenatal care and child health services, with special emphasis on pregnant adolescents.	$478 million FY 1986
Medicaid under Title XIX of the Social Security Act	Finances health care for the poor, including pregnant adolescents and adolescent parents.	$21.7 billion FY 1985
Aid to Families with Dependent Children	Provides financial assistance for eligible adolescent parents and their children.	$7.7 billion FY 1985
Social Services Block Grant through Title XX of the Social Security Act	Provides funds to states that can be used for a variety of social services for pregnant adolescents and adolescent parents.	$2.7 billion FY 1985
National Institute for Child Health and Human Development	Supports behavioral research on teen sex, contraceptive behavior, pregnancy, and parenting.	(not available)
Centers for Disease Control	Collects statistics on sexually transmitted diseases.	(not available)

Compiled from "Adolescent Pregnancy and Childbearing," U.S. Department of Health and Human Services, pp. 1–9.

C. EVALUATION OF FAMILY PLANNING PROGRAMS DESIGNED TO REDUCE TEEN PREGNANCIES AND ABORTIONS

With the tremendous growth in the outlay of federal dollars in family planning for teens, policy makers might expect to see a marked reduction in adolescent pregnancy and abortion. But from 1971 to 1981, when there was a 306 percent increase in federal funding, there was a **48.3 percent increase in teen pregnancies and a 133 percent increase in teen abortions.**[22] This high correlation between federal funding for family planning and intensification of the problems was substantiated in testimony before the U. S. Senate Committee on Labor and Human Resources, as seen in Table 3.[23]

Table 3

Federal Expenditures on Family Planning; Births and Abortions to Women 15–19;
Pregnancies, Births, and Abortions per 1,000 Women 15–19, 1970–81.

Year	Federal expenditures on family planning ($ thousands)	Births to women 15–19	Abortions to women 15–19	Pregnancies per 1,000 women 15–19	Births per 1,000 women 15–19	Abortions per 1,000 women 15–19
1970	—	644,708	—	68.32	68.32	—
1971	80,000	628,000	—	64.66	64.66	—
1972	99,420	616,280	191,000	81.22	62.01	19.22
1973	137,280	604,096	231,890	82.61	59.69	22.91
1974	142,780	595,466	279,700	85.36	58.08	27.28
1975	148,220	582,238	325,780	87.77	56.28	31.49
1976	157,140	558,744	362,680	88.26	53.52	34.74
1977	184,620	559,154	397,720	91.87	53.69	38.19
1978	217,771	543,407	418,790	92.82	52.42	40.40
1979	233,031	549,472	444,600	94.7	52.3	42.4
1980	298,572	552,161	444,800	95.9	53.0	42.7
1981	324,977	527,392	433,000	96.0	52.7	43.3

Source: Figures from 1970–78 from Susan Roylance testimony before U.S. Senate Committee on Labor and Human Resources, March 31, 1981, based on data from National Center for Health Statistics, U.S. Department of Health and Human Services, U.S. Bureau of the Census, and the Alan Guttmacher Institute; figures for 1979–81 from National Center for Health Statistics and the Alan Guttmacher Institute. The figures for family planning expenditures are estimates of certain categories of spending only. While they appear to be internally consistent, they are substantially smaller than other estimates of the same kinds of spending. Used with permission of the American Life League, P.O. Box 1350, Stafford, VA 22554.

Researchers Joseph Olsen and Stan Weed also showed the failure of federal family planning to reduce teen pregnancies and abortions. In their 1986 reports, they concluded:

1. Instead of the expected reduction in teenage pregnancies, greater adolescent **involvement in family planning programs was associated with significantly higher teenage pregnancy rates.**

2. Instead of the expected reduction in teenage abortions, greater adolescent **involvement in family planning programs was associated with significantly higher teenage abortion rates.**

3. The expected net reduction in teenage births was achieved, but due to **a reliance on abortions, not contraceptives.**[24]

Olsen and Weed also questioned the claim by family planners that the increased rates would have been even higher without their services to teens. The findings of Olsen and Weed are depicted in Table 4.

Table 4
Impact of Teenage Family-Planning Programs

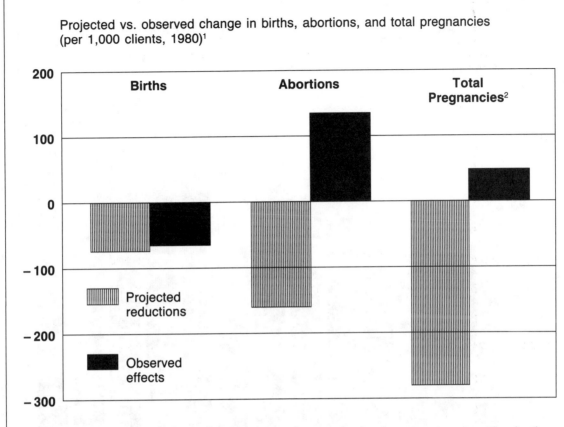

Projected vs. observed change in births, abortions, and total pregnancies
(per 1,000 clients, 1980)[1]

[1] These represent the remaining effects after accounting for race, poverty, urbanization, and residential stability.

[2] Total pregnancies include miscarriages, which are estimated at 20% of births and 10% of abortions.

Sources: Projected reductions (J.D. Forrest, Guttmacher Institute, 1984); Observed effects (Weed, 1989), used with permission.

In 1986, when the U. S. House Select Committee on Children, Youth, and Families investigated the problem of teenage pregnancy, they discovered the same alarming statistics about the increase in teen pregnancies and abortions. The committee minority members (i.e., the Republicans), led by Congressman Dan Coats, expressed concern about the failure of family planning to reduce teen pregnancies and abortion. While family planners were touting the effectiveness of their programs, the committee minority members showed that abortion, not contraceptives, was bringing about the reduction in teen births. To dramatically illustrate their point, the committee presented the bar graph in Table 5.[25]

Table 5
Adolescent Pregnancy Rate and Outcomes, 1970–82

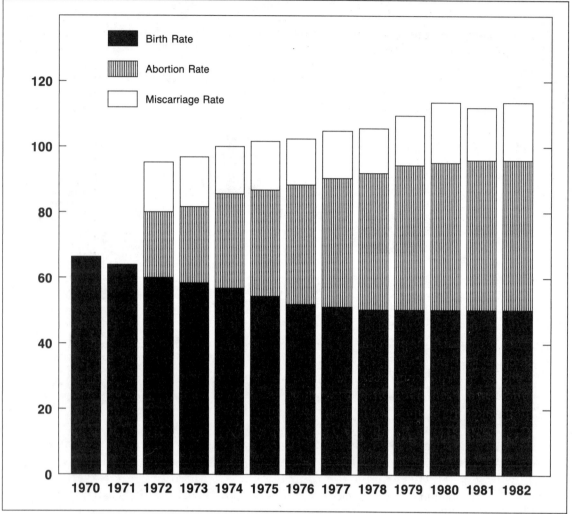

Source: U.S. Select Committee on Children, Youth, and Families, Teen Pregnancy: What Can Be Done? A State-By-State Look, *p. 20.*

NOTE: In the 1980s, the birth rate and pregnancy rate for teens began to decline, as reported in JAMA, 10/16/87, pp. 2067–71.

Since the data in Table 5 were published, more recent statistics have become available. The number of pregnancies per 1,000 females age fifteen to nineteen peaked in 1980 at 111, then dropped to 110 in 1981 and 1982. In 1983, it decreased to 108, showing a general leveling off. The number of live births for women age fifteen to nineteen also decreased in the early 1980s, going from 53 per 1,000 in 1980 to 50.9 in 1984. But the number of abortions remained high.

The correlation between funding for family planning and high levels of teen pregnancies and abortions applies not only to federal programs, but to state programs as well. As revealed in testimony before the U. S. Senate Committee on Labor and Human Resources, those states with the highest expenditures on family planning and with similar socio-demographic characteristics showed the largest increases in abortions and illegitimate births.[26] When comparing selected states to the national average, it becomes glaringly apparent that the rate of teenage pregnancy and abortion closely parallels funding for family planning, as shown in Table 6.[27]

Table 6
Rates of Teenage Pregnancy and Abortion Plus
Unmarried Births for States with FNCC

State	Per capita public expenditures on birth control as a percent of national average, 1980	Teen pregnancy rate as percentage of national average, 1981	Rate of abortion plus unmarried births to teens as percent of national average, 1981
California	227%	133%	150%
Hawaii	170%	122%	134%
Georgia	142%	128%	131%
New York	111%	105%	135%

Source: (As reported in "Teenage Pregnancy: What Comparisons Among States and Countries Show"; Jacqueline Kasun, Ph.D.) Rate for American states computed from data on abortions from U.S. Centers for Disease Control; rates for foreign countries from Elise F. Jones et al, "Teenage Pregnancy in Developed Countries: Determinants and Policy Implications," Family Planning Perspectives, Vol. 17, No. 2, March/April 1985, pp. 53–63; per capita government expenditures on contraceptives and abortions computed from data appearing in Family Planning Perspectives, Vol. 14, No. 4, July/August 1982. Used with permission of the American Life League, P.O. Box 1350, Stafford, VA 22554.

Population researcher Phillips Cutright arrived at the same conclusion regarding funding and teen pregnancy: "We find no evidence that the programs reduced white illegitimacy, because areas with weak programs or no programs at all experience smaller increases or larger declines [in pregnancy] than are found in areas with strong contraceptive programs."[28]

Some advocates of family planning for adolescents (e.g., Zelnik, Kantner, and Zabin) have tried to show there have been benefits from their programs. But as Professor Jacqueline Kasun, a statistician at Humboldt State University, has concluded, statistical errors introduced by small samples are often the basis on which proponents of family planning try to draw a picture of effectiveness. Kasun points out that it is therefore improper to use positive results from such studies to advocate the benefits of family planning programs.[29]

D. ACCESSIBILITY OF FAMILY PLANNING FOR ADOLESCENTS

When asked to explain why their programs have not helped to reduce the teenage pregnancy rate, proponents of family planning have argued that teens lack knowledge of or access to the contraceptive services. For example, in its 1985 report, the Guttmacher Institute cited this as one of the major reasons the U. S. adolescent pregnancy rate was double that of the five other Western countries studied.[30]

However, after an exhaustive review of family planning programs, researchers Olsen and Weed concluded that in the early years of family planning, teen access to family planning services increased dramatically. Table 7 illustrates their point.

Table 7

Year	Number of Teens Served	% of Females Served That Were Under the Age of 20
1970	300,000	23%
1975	1,500,000	30%

Source: Statistics by Olsen and Weed.

Even today, teens have high access to contraceptives. From 1969 to 1987, the number of black teens receiving family planning services tripled, while the number of white teens receiving such services increased seventeenfold! In 1976, only 3 percent of teenagers who did not use contraceptives said it was because they did not know how or where to obtain them.[31] In 1987, Planned Parenthood's own poll showed that only 14 percent of sexually active teens who did not usually use contraceptives attributed their not using protection mainly to a lack of knowledge or access.[32]

Although the proponents of family planning blame the failure of their programs on the lack of access for teens, their own studies reveal the high percentage of teens who are using their programs. The Guttmacher Institute reported that the enrollment in family planning for teens was seven times larger in 1979 than in 1970.[33] Frederick Jaffe, late president of the Institute, estimated that in 1978 less than 20 percent of sexually active teens lacked access to family planning services.[34]

The claim that the failure of family planning programs for teens is due to lack of accessibility therefore seems unfounded.

E. ACCESSIBILITY OF FAMILY PLANNING AND ITS CORRELATE: REPEATED ABORTIONS

Earlier in this report (Section I. C.), it was shown that the teenage abortion rate skyrocketed during the time when family planning programs were growing in scope. But another question about the relationship between family planning and abortion needs to be raised: Is abortion a one-time event for teens facing an unplanned pregnancy, or does it set a pattern for recurring abortions, even when contraceptives are used regularly? A review of studies by family planning groups shows that a repeated occurrence of abortions is taking place in spite of an unprecedented use of contraceptives.

Planned Parenthood studied several family planning services and discovered an increase in premarital pregnancy, even among those teens who always used contraceptives.[35] The *Journal of Biosocial Science* reports that repeat abortion seekers tend to have a better knowledge of contraception and are more regular users of contraceptives than those seeking first abortions.[36] One study by the Centers for Disease Control shows that 50 percent of teenagers who got abortions had been using contraceptives at the time of conception.[37]

Nearly half the 1.1 million teenage pregnancies each year end in abortion,[38] and nearly 10 percent of the teens whose first pregnancy ended in abortion become pregnant again within one year.[39]

One study showed that 71 percent of women who have abortions will have one or more subsequent abortions as well.[40]

These studies show that even when teens regularly use contraceptives, they can still become pregnant, and that the pregnancies often end in abortion. Rather than curtailing sexual activity, many of the same teens re-enter the cycle, resulting in repeated pregnancies and repeated abortions. Notwithstanding, advocates of family planning do not see (or acknowledge) that their programs are failures. In fact, some advocates justify abortion as a necessary means of fertility control when contraceptives fail. As the Guttmacher Institute stated in its 1981 report *Teenage Pregnancy: The Problem That Hasn't Gone Away:*

> We know that many teenagers are making great efforts to prevent pregnancy, that more of them are using contraceptives and using them earlier and more consistently than ever before. Many are doing so successfully. Yet, pregnancy rates among U. S. teenagers are increasing and teenage birth rates, though declining, are still among the highest in the world. **The decline in births is largely contingent on continued access to legal abortions.** (emphasis added)[41]

F. EVALUATION OF FAMILY PLANNING PROGRAMS WITH RELATION TO PROMISCUITY AMONG ADOLESCENTS

Family planning proponents often insist that their programs do not promote promiscuity, and therefore they are not at all responsible for the teen sexuality crisis. Yet, Planned Parenthood listed "universal reproductive freedom" as its major goal in its five-year plan for 1976-80. As early as 1963, then-president of Planned Parenthood Alan Guttmacher (after whom the organization's research arm was named) acknowledged that contraceptive information for teens would bring about an increase in sexual promiscuity.[42]

The inventors of the birth-control pill, on the other hand, had no idea how their creation would contribute to teen sexual activity. In 1977, Dr. Robert Kistner of Harvard Medical School said, "About 10 years ago I declared that the pill would not lead to promiscuity. Well, I was wrong."[43] In 1981, Dr. Min Chueh Chang said, "I personally feel the pill has rather spoiled young people.... It's made them more permissive."[44]

In addition to the inventors of the Pill, other physicians agree that family planning has increased teen sexual activity. In a survey of 400 randomly selected family physicians and psychiatrists, as depicted in Table 8, the majority agreed that the availability of contraceptives has led to increased promiscuity among teens.[45]

Table 8

Has increased availability of contraceptives led to
increased sexual activity among teenagers?

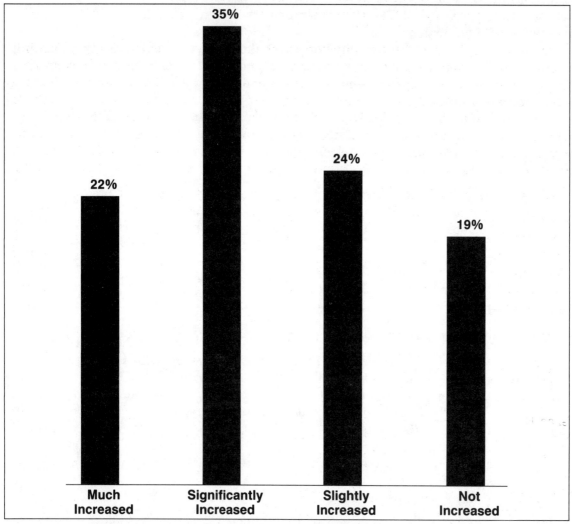

Much Increased	Significantly Increased	Slightly Increased	Not Increased
22%	35%	24%	19%

Source: Medical Aspects of Human Sexuality, *May 1987, p. 147.*

Dr. Frank Furstenberg, professor of sociology at the University of Pennsylvania, said, "Even the most dedicated proponents of widespread contraceptive information availability for teenagers are aware that their efforts may promote sexual activity."[46] The National Research Council also acknowledges, in *Risking the Future,* that contraceptive services to teenagers are associated with increased promiscuity, and that there may even be a causal relationship.[47]

Objective policy makers looking at the history of family planning for teens will probably agree with one of the foremost population control experts, Professor Kingsley Davis of Zero Population Growth, who says:

> The current belief that illegitimacy will be reduced if teenaged girls are given an effective contraceptive is an extension of the same reasoning that created the problem in the first place. It reflects an unwillingness to face problems of social control and social discipline while trusting some technological device to extricate society from its difficulties. The irony is that the illegitimacy rise occurred precisely while contraceptive use was becoming more, rather than less, widespread and respectable.[48]

II. *SCHOOL-BASED CLINICS FOR ADOLESCENTS*

Operating under the assumption that a lack of access to family planning services was a major contributor to the teenage pregnancy rate, family planning proponents developed school-based clinics (SBCs). The basic intention of SBCs is to increase access to health care services, bringing them directly onto school campuses, particularly in low-income, minority neighborhoods. Teenagers will thus be able to receive services at low or no cost, at convenience to the client, and at a crucial intervention stage. Also, clinic advocates believe that by having close supervision of teens taking contraceptives, they will help teens to become regular, not sporadic, users.

Some of the goals of SBCs are commendable (e.g., to help a pregnant teen stay in school and not become a dropout). The compassionate undertones of the SBC movement have caused leaders in underprivileged neighborhoods to pay close attention to the appeals. But a review of the history, cost, and questionable effectiveness of SBCs will show that policy makers would be wise to avoid implementing these programs in their schools, particularly because family planning is often a hidden agenda for SBC advocates.

A. BACKGROUND INFORMATION ABOUT SCHOOL-BASED CLINICS

The first SBC opened in Dallas in 1970 and was sponsored by the University of Texas Health Science Center. Three years later, a clinic was opened at Mechanic Arts High School in St. Paul, Minnesota, sponsored by the Maternal and Infant Care Program of the St. Paul Ramsey Hospital. Two additional clinics were opened in St. Paul schools. As of 1987, there were at least 61 known clinics in 27 cities across 17 states. Another 198 are under consideration at the time of this writing.[49]

The major national organization promoting SBCs is the Center for Population Options (CPO). The Center has developed the Support Center for School-Based Clinics, which puts out reports, publishes books, holds training sessions, furnishes consultants, and gives advice.[50] Quite often, proponents of SBCs in a local community interact closely with representatives from Planned Parenthood, the March of Dimes, the Children's Defense Fund, the Urban League, the YWCA, and other groups concerned about the problem of teenage pregnancy.[51] Planned Parenthood president Faye Wattleton strongly supports SBCs. In 1986, when accepting the award for Humanist of the Year, she declared, "Easier access to contraception must be another priority—access without any barriers. We must establish more school-based health clinics that provide contraceptives as part of general health care."[52]

The CPO teaches local supporters of SBCs how to implement these services. The CPO's advice includes emphasizing health care needs while **downplaying the issue of family planning,** setting up an advisory committee only of those who support SBCs, and cultivating the press.[53]

The strategy is usually effective in circumventing opposition. When parents and other people discover that a clinic is being implemented in their community, their strongest objection is to the family planning component. Usually, proponents reassure opponents that the SBC is designed to meet important unmet needs, and that family planning will not be provided or, if provided, will play a minor role. But the CPO's survey shows that **family planning is a vital factor in SBCs.** See Table 9 for some of the survey results.

Table 9
SBCs and Contraceptives

80% of clinics dispense contraceptive prescriptions

50% of clinics refer for contraceptive prescriptions

50% of clinics dispense contraceptives on campus

NOTE: The sum of these percentages exceeds 100 because some clinics provide one or more of the services listed.

The CPO also said that "by definition, all of the clinics are involved in family planning."[54] The Robert Wood Johnson Foundation, one of the largest sources of funding for SBCs, **requires** that family planning services be included in order for a school to be eligible for funding.

When questioned about the cost of school-based clinics, advocates say that private foundation grants are available to underwrite the projects. The Robert Wood Johnson, Rockefeller, Ford, Mellon, Hewlett, Carnegie, Kaiser, and MacArthur foundations are in fact some of the major sources of funding for SBCs.[55] And when training sessions are held in key cities of the country, advocates of SBCs teach communities how to apply for these grants.[56]

According to the Support Center for School-Based Clinics, the cost of clinics ranges from about $25,000 to $400,000 per clinic annually.[57] A proposed clinic in North Carolina suggests that an average annual cost of $79,000 would be spent on a single clinic to serve about six teens per day. That translates to about $73.88 per student each day served,[58] a surprisingly sizable fee in comparison to the rates at private clinics.

Naturally, most local supporters of SBCs welcome foundation grants to cover these enormous expenses. But many people do not realize that when the grants run out (usually within three years), the school district and local community must assume the cost. At that stage, a heavy tax burden often causes local officials to look to their states for help. Before local officials ever get in such a predicament, however, they should realize that most of the services of SBCs are already available in their communities through family planning clinics, municipal hospitals, and private physicians. When school officials realize the potential liability placed upon them by having a SBC on their campus, they often recognize they are unprepared to assume the additional responsibility.

Besides the cost and liability accompanying SBCs, policy makers need to question whether or not such services are effective in reducing the teenage pregnancy rate.

B. REPORTS ON SPECIFIC SCHOOL-BASED CLINICS

In recent years, advocates of SBCs have cited three cases in which they claim their services have lowered the adolescent pregnancy rate. But close analysis shows the studies are flawed.

1. The St. Paul Case

Advocates of SBCs refer to St. Paul schools as an example of how the program helped to reduce the birth rate in the 1970s. Indicating a pregnancy decrease of 40 percent and a birth decline of 23 percent from 1973 to 1976, the St. Paul results are hailed as a reason to promote this type of service across the country.[59] However, there are four reasons to question the findings:

- Even Douglas Kirby, formerly of the national Support Center for SBCs, says, "Most of the evidence for the success of that program is based upon the clinic's own records and/or the staff's knowledge of births among students. Thus the data undoubtedly do not include all births."[60]

- Advocates of the St. Paul clinic fail to take into account the number of pregnancies that ended in abortion. At a national conference on SBCs, it was acknowledged that "whether the decline [in teen births] was due to a decrease in the number of pregnancies or to an increase in reliance on abortion cannot be discerned."[61]

- The studies fail to point out that the student population at the school declined, a factor not weighed in the reports. In 1977, the student population was 1,268. By 1979, the enrollment was down some 25 percent to 948. A similar reduction of 25 percent in reported births would not be unexpected, given the decline in the student population.[62]

- Researcher Marie Dietz notes, "The widely publicized findings of the teenage contraceptive clinic which supposedly showed a drop in the birth rate are simply not supported by the data presented in the report."[63]

2. The Baltimore Case

In 1985, advocates of SBCs claimed that the Johns Hopkins Pregnancy Prevention Program had helped to reduce teenage pregnancies at two Baltimore schools.[64] Professor Jacqueline Kasun has challenged those findings, however. In a letter to Kasun, the superintendent of public instruction in Baltimore stated that the questionnaire on which the advocates' conclusions were drawn had not been administered in the schools, and as a result, the school was investigating the project.[65]

But even if questionnaires were correctly administered, there remain serious flaws in the Baltimore claims:

- The study does not take into account the number of girls who dropped out of school due to pregnancy. There was a 33 percent decline in the number of girls surveyed between the first and last surveys done in the study, reflecting the fact that the school with the SBC had a dropout rate three times higher than that of the schools without clinics. Investigators estimated that as many as half of such dropouts may be due to pregnancy. The omission from the study sample of the girls who dropped out due to pregnancy casts serious doubt on the SBC's conclusion that its program reduced teen sex and pregnancy rates.[66]

- The SBC's claim of a delay in sexual activity and a reduction in pregnancy is based on limited sampling. The first questionnaire surveyed only 96 of the 1033 girls in the program, and presumably it would have been easy to survey many more. The limited nature of the sample raises the question of how those surveyed were selected for the study.[67]

- Advocates of the Baltimore clinic calculated pregnancy rates as percentages of the sexually active and did not include all girls exposed to the clinic program. This approach means that even if pregnancy rose as a result of the clinic program, if it rose less rapidly than sexual activity, it would appear to have declined. Thus, two failures could be made to look like a success. The advocates' description of their statistical methods strongly suggests this is just what happened.[68]

   This statistical phenomenon (whereby two failures combined look like a success) occasionally occurs in the reporting of teenage pregnancy rates. For example, using data from 1974 to 1980 nationwide, the United States Department of Health and Human Services reported the same occurrence—pregnancies among all fifteen- to nineteen-year-olds increased by 8.2 percent. But if shown as the percentage of sexually active teens only, then pregnancies appeared to **decrease** by 5.7 percent.[69]

- The advocates of the clinic give percentages rather than numbers in the categories studied. In this case, very few students were studied.[70]

- The advocates did not have sufficient control over all predictive variables. The control group did not have a comparable population, nor the same curricula as the students at the clinic. Nor can the transiency of the inner-city student population at the selected site be compared elsewhere.[71]

- The study took into account very short-term results, not long-range effects.[72]

- The Baltimore student population and other variables were unique. Therefore, the study cannot be replicated elsewhere.[73]

3. The Chicago Case

In June 1985, Chicago's DuSable High School opened a school-based clinic. Television and newspaper reports have touted the effectiveness of the clinic in reducing teen pregnancies despite the fact that no records of pregnancies were kept before the clinic opened.[74] Unlike the St. Paul and Baltimore cases, there have not yet been any official publications by researchers regarding the effectiveness of the program.

The uniqueness of the Chicago situation is that it has brought about an unprecedented backlash by citizens in the predominantly black neighborhood. Parents, students, pastors, and other community leaders have formed the Pro-Life/Pro-Family Coalition to get such clinics removed from their schools. The Coalition has brought a lawsuit against the school district. The charge pending at the time of this writing is that the state legislature does not explicitly empower the schools to operate medical clinics and that schools only have powers delegated to them explicitly by the legislature.[75]

These three cases call into question the supposed effectiveness of school-based clinics. Douglas Kirby, former director of research for the Center for Population Options, admitted that their services demonstrate "no measurable impact" on teen pregnancy rates. Kirby reported these results in a workshop titled "Effectiveness of SBCs" at the annual meeting of the National Family Planning and Reproductive Health Association. Despite the realization of the failure of SBCs to reduce the teenage pregnancy rate, however, the CPO will continue to promote them.[76]

Given the lack of demonstrated effectiveness of SBCs, however, policy makers may agree with Myron Lieberman, writing in the *Journal of Family and Culture:* "The educational landscape reveals a mindless commitment of public school resources to the solution of social problems that are beyond their influence. In the long run, the waste of resources, substantial as it is, may be less important than the loss of respect for public schools engendered by such misguided efforts."[77]

III. *COMPREHENSIVE SEX EDUCATION*

During the 1960s, as the fear of overpopulation became prevalent, family planning groups not only advocated the federal funding of adolescent contraceptive programs, but they also proposed sex education as a means to reduce teenage pregnancy. In *Implementing DHEW Policy on Family Planning* in 1966, the Department of Health, Education, and Welfare stated that its sex information was designed as a means of effective fertility control, especially among minorities. Planned Parenthood and Sex Information and Education Council of the United States (SIECUS) said that they had as their duty the changing of people's values regarding sexuality and the reduction of fertility.[78]

Whereas family planning for married adults became an acceptable phenomenon in the 1960s, sex education was received with more reluctance. Contemporary sex educators have blamed society's apprehension about allowing sexuality to be discussed in the classroom for contributing to the problem of teen pregnancy.[79] Their cause received strong impetus from the Guttmacher Institute's much-publicized 1985 report.

However, considering that family planning and school-based clinics have not yet been shown to be effective in reducing teen pregnancy, policy makers should question the effectiveness of comprehensive sex education, as well. A close examination of its various aspects will show not only that it is a failure, but that it can also produce serious harm to young people.

A. WHAT IS COMPREHENSIVE SEX EDUCATION?

In the 1950s, Sweden adopted a form of sex education that served as the prototype for the Western world. The Swedish approach, coinciding with its culture's permissive views toward sex, was based on the premise that teenage sex was inevitable, that educators should take a neutral stand on morality, that schools should openly discuss sexual matters, and that educators should teach students about contraception.[80] The same approach, though not directly attributed to Sweden, was eventually adopted in the United States within fifteen years. The method has been given various names: "sex education," "progressive sex education," "contemporary sex education," "modern sex education," "contraceptive sex education," "values-neutral sex education," and "comprehensive sex education." Recently, "family life education" has been adopted because it has a more favorable connotation than "sex education."

A Louis Harris poll on teenage sexuality commissioned by Planned Parenthood helps clarify what is meant by "comprehensive sex education." The poll used six criteria to determine whether or not a person had had a course in "comprehensive sex education." If the course contained four of the six elements, it could be classified as comprehensive:

1. biological facts about reproduction;
2. talk about coping with your sexual development;
3. information about different kinds of birth control;
4. information about preventing sexual abuse;
5. facts about abortion; and
6. facts about where to get contraceptives.[81]

B. PREVALENCE OF COMPREHENSIVE SEX EDUCATION IN THE SCHOOLS

Although the Guttmacher Institute claims that sex education is not prevalent in the United States, numerous studies show it is widespread. One study found that 40 percent of all teens have had sex education, while another report gives a statistic as high as 75 percent.[82] Different studies produce different figures, but they all confirm that sex education is common across the country.

A 1982 survey of 179 school districts in large cities showed that 75 percent provide varying degrees of sex education at the secondary level, and 66 percent provide it at the elementary level.[83] A 1984 study showed that 60 percent of women and 52 percent of men now in their twenties had taken a sex education course by age nineteen.[84]

The 1986 Louis Harris poll showed that of all teens surveyed who had some form of sex education, 60 percent indicated it was "comprehensive" in nature.[85]

AIDS education is also spreading in schools across the country, particularly in response to then Surgeon General C. Everett Koop's call for such programs. In December 1987, the Council of Chief State School Officers (CCSSO) conducted an AIDS Education Needs Assessment. Released on July 8, 1988, the results showed that twenty-eight states already have a state policy or law on AIDS education, and twenty-four have mandatory AIDS education in public schools. More than half the states surveyed (twenty-eight) already have a state curriculum or curriculum guide, and eight states and Washington, D.C., have a mandatory curriculum. All the states indicated that abstinence is discussed in their AIDS education; twenty-four discuss condom usage; twenty discuss safe sex; and fifteen discuss homosexuality.[86]

While it may appear that abstinence is the most frequent message conveyed in these states, the discussion of condom usage and safe sex suggests that most states are following the value-neutral approach in their AIDS programs. Selected states have mandated sex and AIDS education laws that do not follow the safe sex approach but emphasize abstinence and warn of the failure of condoms. (Refer to section V. A. 4. of this report for a list of states which passed abstinence legislation in 1988.)

Tables 10-12 below show the status of AIDS education as of December 1987, compiled by the CCSSO.

Thus, numerous studies confirm the prevalence, not shortage, of sex education courses in the United States. This finding should cast serious doubt on the Guttmacher Institute's claim that the teen pregnancy rate is due to a lack of programs in the schools.

In spite of this prevalence of sex education, Planned Parenthood has targeted various states so that schools would be mandated to teach comprehensive sex education. In its most recent "Five-Year Plan," Planned Parenthood Federation of America commits to increase to fifteen the number of states with mandatory K—12 sexuality educational curricula. To accomplish this goal, the organization has devised a "tiered" strategy. Tier one states (including Connecticut, Nevada, Oregon, Texas, Vermont, Virginia, and Wisconsin) are the highest priority. As of 1988, Planned Parenthood has been successful in getting Nevada to mandate sex education, and has helped to get Virginia's state department of education to establish new K—12 guidelines. Besides success in the tier one states, Planned Parenthood has targeted eight states in tier two, and the remaining states in tier three. As states are considering how to resolve the problem of teenage pregnancy, they tend to be strongly influenced by the Planned Parenthood concept of what sex education should be.[87]

Table 10
24 States Have Mandatory AIDS Education in Schools

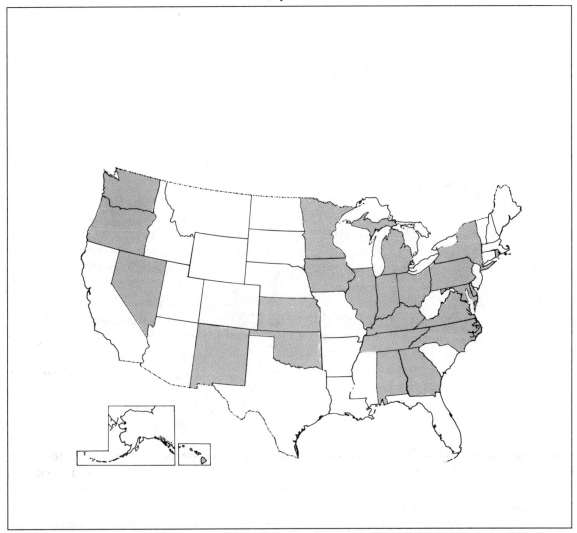

Based on "AIDS Education Needs Assessment" (Dec. 1987). Conducted by the Council of Chief State School Officers, cited in The Education Reporter, *August 1988. Used with permission of* The Education Reporter.

C. DOES COMPREHENSIVE SEX EDUCATION HELP TO REDUCE THE TEENAGE PREGNANCY RATE?

While advocates of comprehensive sex education are calling for expansion of their programs, many are also admitting their programs have failed. In 1981, researchers Zelnik and Kantner acknowledged that there was an "almost total absence of evidence" of any benefits of sex education.[88] Planned Parenthood printed a review of studies claiming that sex education was beneficial, but the same studies show that the teenage promiscuity and pregnancy rates had increased, not decreased, during the time span in question.[89]

The National Education Association, which promotes K–12 sex education, admits that "while many feel that sex-education programs are necessary to halt the spread of venereal disease and the rise of illegitimate children, **there is as yet only meager evidence that such programs reduce the incidence of these phenomena**" (emphasis added).[90]

Table 11
8 States Have Mandatory AIDS Curriculum

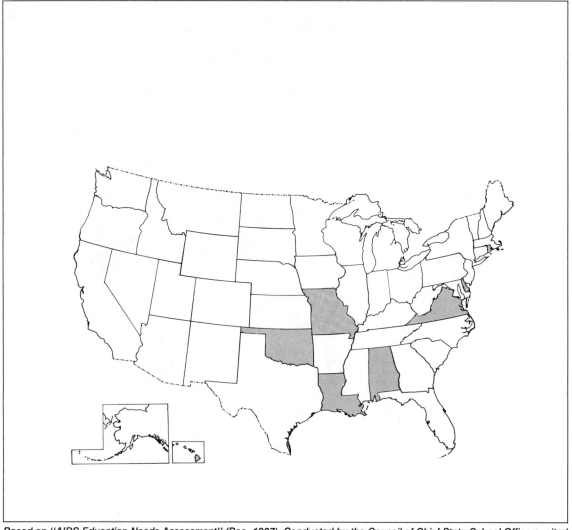

Based on "AIDS Education Needs Assessment" (Dec. 1987). Conducted by the Council of Chief State School Officers, cited in The Education Reporter, *August 1988. Used with permission of* The Education Reporter.

Douglas Kirby, former director of research for the Center for Population Options and an advocate of school-based clinics, acknowledges: "Past studies of sex education suggest several conclusions. They indicate that sex education programs can increase knowledge, but they also indicate that most programs have relatively little impact on values. . . . **programs certainly do not appear to have as dramatic an impact on behavior as professionals once had hoped**" (emphasis added).[91]

In the March 1989 issue of *Pediatrics,* Dr. James W. Stout reviewed five studies on the effects of sex education and concluded that sex education has had little impact on altering sexual activity, promoting the use of birth control, or lowering teenage pregnancy. In another report, Dr. Stout compared the failure of sex education to the failure of cigarette campaigns, saying, "People can have the information regarding their health, but it doesn't automatically translate into their behavior. A good example would be the ill health effects of cigarette smoking, which it's probably safe to say most smokers are aware of, and yet they still smoke."[92]

A study of sex education by Johns Hopkins University draws the same conclusion about the failure:

The final result to emerge from the analysis is that neither pregnancy education nor contraceptive education exerts any significant effect on the risk of premarital

Table 12
At What Level Is AIDS Education Introduced?

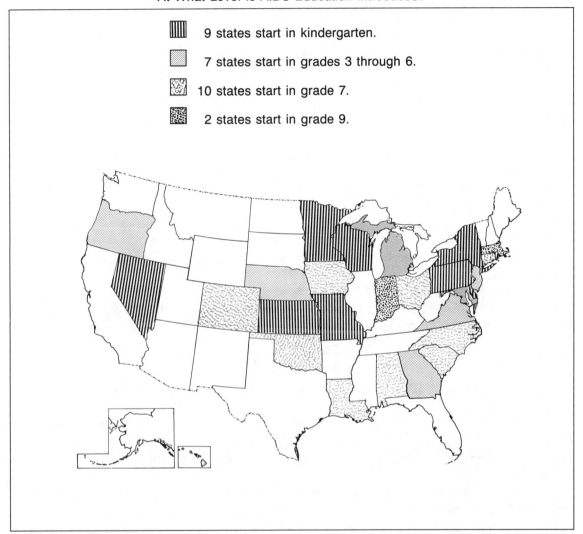

IIII	9 states start in kindergarten.
▫	7 states start in grades 3 through 6.
▨	10 states start in grade 7.
▓	2 states start in grade 9.

Based on "AIDS Education Needs Assessment" (Dec. 1987). Conducted by the Council of Chief State School Officers, cited in The Education Reporter, *August 1988. Used with permission of* The Education Reporter.

pregnancy among sexually active teenagers—**a finding that calls into question the argument that formal sex education is an effective tool for reducing adolescent pregnancy.**[93]

Thus, with some advocates of comprehensive sex education admitting their own programs are unsuccessful, community decision makers should consider the findings carefully before they implement the same types of programs.

D. COMPREHENSIVE SEX EDUCATION AND SEXUAL ACTIVITY

In October 1986, then Surgeon General Koop issued a statement about the danger of AIDS and called for K–12 sex education to help reduce the spread of AIDS. Proponents of comprehensive sex education seized Dr. Koop's statement as an endorsement of their programs. But after seeing the explicitness of many classroom materials, Dr. Koop, along with then Secretary of Education William Bennett, stated his view of what constitutes appropriate sex education. And their philosophy is diametrically opposed to the approach of comprehensive sex educators.[94]

What contemporary educators fail to realize is that the boldness of their approach seems to desensitize young people and inclines them to become more permissive. That finding goes all the way back to the very first sex education program in the Western world—the Swedish approach. In 1956, when Sweden mandated sex education, **the illegitimacy rate, which had been declining, rose for every school age group, except the older ones, who did not receive the special education.**[95]

The same can be said about sex education in American schools. Bruno Bettleheim, quoted in *Psychology Today,* has observed that the approach in schools should be **"implicated in the increase in teenage sex and teenage pregnancies"** (emphasis added).[96]

Researchers Marsiglio and Mott confirm the view, showing that **sex education is associated with an increase in sexual activity** among fifteen- and sixteen-year-olds. They admit that a course in sex education may lead to an increase in regular contraceptive use, but the net impact of these two factors on premarital pregnancy is modest.[97]

A review of thirty-three studies of sex education showed that there were gains in sexual knowledge but **shifts toward more liberal sexual attitudes, which lead to promiscuity.**[98]

Summing it all up, Furstenberg reported that **"even the most dedicated proponents of widespread contraceptive information availability for teenagers are aware that their efforts may promote sexual activity"** (emphasis added).[99]

E. COMPREHENSIVE SEX EDUCATION AND ADOLESCENT EMOTIONAL RESPONSES

Comprehensive sex education has also been correlated with an increase in emotional problems for adolescents. Dr. Myre Sim, professor of psychiatry at the University of Ottawa, has described the approach used by contemporary sex educators as "bad education."[100]

Dr. Melvin Anchell, author of numerous books on human sexuality, explains the reason for the correlation:

Typical sex education courses are almost perfect recipes for producing personality problems and even perversions later in life. . . . Sex education programs from kindergarten through high school continuously downgrade the affectionate, monogamous nature of human sexuality. Sex education, whether purposeful or not, desensitizes students to the spiritual qualities of human sexuality.

Attributing emotional instability partly to progressive sex education, Dr. Anchell further criticizes contemporary programs:

In the past twenty years or so, the number of adolescents admitted to hospitals for depression has tripled and adolescent suicide has increased by 200%. Some of the blame for this decline in adolescent mental health must fall on the carnal attitudes toward sex, as well as premature sexual activity, encouraged by contemporary sex education.[101]

The minority members of the U. S. House Committee on Children, Youth, and Families made the same point in their report, *Teen Pregnancy: What Is Being Done? A State-by-State Look:*

Progressively over the past 25 years we have as a nation decided that it is easier to give children pills than to teach them respect for sex and marriage. Today we are seeing the results of that decision not only in increased pregnancy rates but in increased rates of drug abuse, venereal disease, suicide, and other forms of self-destructive behavior.[102]

Contemporary sex educators and family planners often fail to see that teens who have engaged in sex and come to their clinics have emotional or personal problems, and that their request for contraceptives is actually a cry for help with their personal needs. As Dr. Jerome Shen observes, "Many adolescents who ask for contraceptives are really asking for help in coping with sexuality and other problems." The adolescent's request for contraceptives does not indicate maturity, and Dr. Shen goes on to point out that these adolescents should **not** be placed on contraceptives.[103]

Josh McDowell, speaker, author, and developer of the national "Why Wait?" program, has pinpointed the cause of the teenage crisis, saying, "I don't believe we've had a sexual revolution. Rather, I believe we have experienced a revolution in search of intimacy."[104]

Until educators realize that teens need intimacy, not more sexual gratification, they will continue to find that their approach worsens the problem and adds to the emotional instability of teens.

F. COMPREHENSIVE SEX EDUCATION AND BIOLOGICAL FACTS

In the 1980s, decision-making models served as the framework for most sex education courses. The assumption underlying this approach is that when presented with all the facts regarding sexual matters, teenagers will be able to make responsible choices. But educators following this approach often present only the pros of sexual involvement, not the cons, neglecting to include important information regarding contraceptive failure rates, the side effects of contraceptive drugs, the myths about safe sex, and the harms of abortion. In doing so, educators have skewed their decision-making models, often giving teens the impression that responsible choices equate with contraceptive usage and continuing sex, not abstinence.

1. The Failure Rate for Teens Using the Pill

One of the items not covered in decision-making models is the failure rate for teens using the Pill. The Pill is considered the most effective contraceptive on the market, and educators usually teach that it has only a 1 percent failure rate when used regularly. However, several studies show the failure rate is higher.

As early as 1973, a study reported in Planned Parenthood's *Family Planning Perspective* showed that teens who regularly use the Pill experience a pregnancy rate four to five times higher than that for older women using the pill.[105] In 1976, another study in *Family Planning Perspective* showed that teens who regularly use the Pill experience a 5.8 percent pregnancy rate.[106]

In 1986, yet another study in *Family Planning Perspective* revealed that while the failure rate for all married women was 2.9 percent, the failure rate for married women under twenty was 4.7 percent. The same study showed that single women under eighteen who use the Pill to "delay" pregnancy have a 4.5 percent failure rate, and those single women under eighteen who use the Pill to "prevent" pregnancy have an 11 percent failure rate.[107]

A study by Cornell University reported in the *Journal of Adolescent Health Care* in 1986 showed that among teenagers who used the Pill with a high rate of compliance, 18 percent reported at least one pregnancy within the first year of use.[108] In 1982, a study in *Family Planning Perspective* showed that the average combined pregnancy rate for teens using contraceptives (of various types, not just the Pill) with a high rate of compliance was 9.9 percent to 13 percent annually.[109] These are the *best* results to be expected from teens who *regularly* use the Pill. Since most teens use the Pill *irregularly,* much higher pregnancy rates can be anticipated.

Besides the fact that teenagers can become pregnant even when using the Pill, educators need to realize that lack of compliance is a probable behavior to anticipate from adolescents. Among the most formidable reasons for lack of compliance are risk taking, denial, guilt associated with deliberate planning, shame if caught, and forgetfulness. Even when females take the Pill daily, the low-dosage pills must be taken at the same time every day to be effective.

2. The Side Effects of the Pill

One study has shown there are common side effects for teens on the Pill, and these are often contributing reasons why teens don't use it as prescribed. Among the effects are weight gain (22%), menstrual problems (18%), nausea (16%), headaches (10%), and abdominal pain (10%).[110] Less common but more serious side effects (e.g., blood clotting) can occur, particularly if the Pill user is a smoker.[111]

Before issuing the Pill, most physicians agree that a medical history and physical exam should be completed on a patient.[112] But, because teens usually do not know about their family's medical history, and because they can receive contraceptives without parental consent, some unscreened teens may be at greater risk than others for adverse drug reactions when they get on the Pill.

3. The Prevalence and Dangers of Sexually Transmitted Disease

According to the Centers for Disease Control, each day 33,000 people contract a sexually transmitted disease. That equates to 12 million cases a year, up from 4 million in 1980. At this rate, one in four Americans between fifteen and fifty-five eventually will acquire a STD. Millions will suffer from infection, pain, infertility, and miscarriages because of these diseases, many of which (e.g., Chlamydia) were unknown until recently and are still hard to detect.[113]

While the STD rate is severe for the population as a whole, the rate in the sixteen-to twenty-year-old age group is three times that of the general population.[114] For example, Chlamydia has become the most commonly diagnosed STD, and among sexually active teens, its prevalence may be as high as 30 percent. Its incidence in teens can be called epidemic.[115]

Other STDs are also increasing among teens. Cervical cancer, now classified as a STD, is a problem especially among young teens. A British report has shown that sexually active females under the age of sixteen are twice as likely to get cervical cancer as those who began sexual activity at seventeen.[116] The reason is that younger teens have more cervical tissue at risk, and such tissue is in the transformation stage. When exposed to human papilloma virus (HPV) from male sex partners, the cervical cells in early adolescents tend to mutate more easily.[117] The prevalence among sexually active teens is estimated to be 11–22 percent.[118]

Besides the serious effects associated with particular STDs, other complications can occur. Girls with STDs sometimes develop pelvic inflammatory disease.[119] And people with certain types of STDs are more susceptible to infection with the AIDS virus.[120]

A report released at the 1988 International Conference on AIDS shows that prostitutes on the Pill have a greater incidence of AIDS than prostitutes not on the Pill. This raises the possibility that the Pill, when used by sexually active women with multiple partners, can produce a condition that assists the entry of the virus into the bloodstream.[121]

4. The Myth of Safe Sex

The notion of "safe sex" became popular in the late 1980s, and condom usage has been promoted as a means of preventing sexually transmitted diseases. Former Surgeon

24

General Koop has said, "The country has become involved in 'condom mania.' I don't feel particularly happy about the role I've played in that. Condoms are a last resort."[122]

There are numerous reasons to say that safe sex is a myth. Perhaps the most dramatic study of the failure of condoms to reduce the spread of AIDS appeared in a 1987 issue of the *Journal of the American Medical Association*. Researchers studied AIDS transmission among spouses in which one partner was infected with the virus. The results showed that the rate of transmission between couples using condoms was 17 percent over a relatively short time (eighteen months). There was no apparent seroconversion (transmission of the disease) among the couples who abstained from sexual intercourse.[123]

Many physicians are now calling for condom advocates to reexamine their position. An interesting example shows that proponents of safe sex themselves are questioning how safe it is. Dr. Theresa Crenshaw, immediate past president of the American Association of Sex Education, Counselors, and Therapists, recalls the way her colleagues responded to a question about condom usage:

> On June 19, 1987, I gave a lecture on AIDS to 800 sexologists at the World Congress of Sexologie in Heidelberg. Most of them recommended condoms to their clients and students. I asked them if they had available the partner of their dreams, and knew that person carried the virus, would they have sex, depending on a condom for protection? No one raised their hand. After a long delay, one timid hand surfaced from the back of the room. I told them that it was irresponsible to give advice to others that they would not follow themselves. The point is, putting a mere balloon between a healthy body and a deadly disease is not safe.[124]

Health care officials are questioning the ethics of advocating and testing safe sex, particularly among high risk groups. The federal government has cut off funds for a UCLA study because the AIDS infection rate among Los Angeles homosexuals is so high that condoms may be incapable of providing reliable protection to study participants. Dr. Jeffrey Perlman, project officer for the UCLA grant, said, "What has happened in the last two years is that gays in Los Angeles became supersaturated with the virus so that to [go ahead with] this study [would mean] there is going to be a large proportion of the recruits who would have become infected. On that basis, it really came to an ethical issue." Federal officials say that five U. S. cities have especially high infection rates among gays, and that condom usage in those places has been seriously compromised. The cities are Los Angeles, San Francisco, New York, Miami, and Washington, D.C.[125]

Across the country, schools and health agencies have taken seriously the responsibility to inform the public about AIDS. (Refer to section III. B. to see which states have implemented AIDS education.) However, in the selection of appropriate materials, many decision makers have raised important questions about whether safe sex is a responsible policy to advocate. In response to questions, the U. S. Department of Education put together a paper entitled "Will 'Safe Sex' Education Effectively Combat AIDS?" It also prepared *AIDS and the Education of Our Children: Guide for Parents and Teachers*. The former refutes the notion of safe sex, and the latter teaches the importance of abstinence.[126]

Among the data that dispel safe sex is the fact that condoms have an overall 10 percent failure rate to prevent pregnancy,[127] and they have an even higher failure rate in preventing the spread of the AIDS virus, evidently because the AIDS virus is so small.[128] When condoms are not used in a highly disciplined way, the failure rate increases, which accounts for why teenagers have a higher condom failure rate (18%).[129]

Furthermore, condoms are not designed to be used in all circumstances. They have a greater likelihood to fail in anal sex.[130] Also, they do not protect people with minor wounds in the pubic area.[131]

While the Food and Drug Administration (FDA) previously allowed lots of up to four condoms per thousand that leak to be acceptable for public sale,[132] it has had to issue recalls in some circumstances. In one investigation the FDA found about 20 percent of the batches to be unsuitable.[133] Now the FDA allows less than three per thousand to be defective.

While condoms might help to reduce (though not eliminate) the spread of STDs, there are nevertheless problems in advocating their usage. Their availability and the widespread knowledge about how to use them do not ensure usage by persons of high risk.[134] For all these reasons, many physicians and public health officials are redefining safe sex to mean premarital abstinence, marital fidelity, and total abstinence among infected persons.[135]

5. Abortion and Its Sequelae

Of the 1.1 million teen pregnancies annually, 40–50 percent end in abortion.[136] Often, the abortion seeker is unaware of the potential physical and psychological consequences of abortion. In part, this may be due to what students have been taught about abortion in the classroom. In comprehensive sex education, abortion is viewed as an integral subject, and it is often described as a perfectly safe procedure.[137] Major medical journals, however, offer studies to show that abortion is not hazard-free.

In 1983, the *New England Journal of Medicine* published an article titled "The Risks Associated With Teenage Abortion." The authors reported that though teenagers have lower rates of morbidity and mortality from abortion than older women, young teenagers have an increased risk of cervical injury during suction-curettage abortion, which is the predominant procedure performed during the first trimester. The authors noted:

> Even when we controlled for parity, type of anesthesia, and the method of dilation, the increased risk of cervical injury in young teenagers persisted. Other investigators have also found that young nulliparous women had higher rates of cervical trauma. These findings cause concern because cervical injury in initial unplanned pregnancies may predispose young women to adverse outcomes in future planned pregnancies.[138]

Though improved abortion techniques have helped to reduce cervical injury, the harms are nevertheless significant for young adolescents.

In a 1982 *Science* journal, studies were cited suggesting that induced abortion can result in a threefold higher ratio of miscarriage in future desired pregnancies.[139]

Another potential complication correlated to abortion is ectopic pregnancies (in which gestation occurs outside the uterus). The number of ectopic pregnancies in the United States has increased almost threefold from 1970 to 1980,[140] during the time in which abortion became legalized. Though the death rate from ectopic pregnancies has fallen dramatically during this same time span, it still accounts for about 10 percent of all maternal mortality. It also adds to an increased likelihood of future compromised fertility, increased future miscarriages, and recurrent ectopic pregnancies. Though there are several contributing factors to ectopic pregnancies, abortion is cited among the nine risk factors associated with the increased rates.[141]

In addition to cervical injury, complications in future planned pregnancies, and ectopic pregnancies, teenagers who abort are also at risk for other problems. Studies have shown that a woman is at lower risk of developing breast cancer if she gives birth at a young age, but only if she has a full-term pregnancy. When first pregnancies terminate within the first four months, there appears to be an **increased** risk of breast cancer. A Los Angeles study found that in certain circumstances, the risk of breast cancer in young women more than doubled if they had had an abortion (either induced or spontaneous).[142]

Besides potential physical problems, there are possible psychological consequences of abortion. Postabortion syndrome affects from 7 to 41 percent of all women who aborted.[143] One of the reasons postabortion syndrome has not received widespread discussion is that there is no systematic review of the literature on the psychological impact of abortion.

Lyons, et al, under a grant from the Office of Population Affairs, conducted a comprehensive search for all abortion studies published in journals over the past two decades, doing a computer search of six scientific databases. The review produced a total of sixty-one quantitative studies. The authors of 62 percent of the articles concluded that abortion had no negative psychological consequences, 17 percent found that abortion did have negative effects, and 21 percent were neutral or cited mixed effects.

Though these statistics would appear to suggest that postabortion syndrome is not prevalent, a closer review of the studies reveals some methodological shortcomings. Lyons and his associates discovered that few studies had adequate control groups or used reliable assessments, no standards existed for studying the impact of abortion over time, and controlled studies of abortion lack sufficient statistical power to detect significant effects. Understandably, then, the majority of studies detected no psychosocial effects of abortion. Lyons and his associates call for further, careful research in order to accurately detect the impact of abortion on individuals.[144]

In January 1989, then Surgeon General C. Everett Koop arrived at the same conclusion and asked that there be a well-designed study to test for the psychological effects of abortion.

Summary About the Lack of Facts

Though contemporary sex educators say they present a well-balanced, decision-making model, it is highly unlikely that teens will be able to make informed choices without the necessary data regarding contraceptive failure, its side effects, sexually transmitted diseases, the myth of safe sex, and the effects of abortion. Professor Jacqueline Kasun, who has written many articles on contemporary sex education, observes:

> It may come as a surprise to other parents, as it did to me, that the contemporary sex education movement does not focus primarily on the biological aspects of sex. The movement leaders and disciples are not biologists but mainly psychologists, sociologists, and "health educators." Their principal concerns are less with the physiology of procreation and inheritance than with "sexuality," a very broad field of interest running the gamut from personal hygiene to the population question, but largely concerned with attitudes and "values clarification" rather than with biological facts.[145]

G. COMPREHENSIVE SEX EDUCATION AND COHABITATION

In value-free sex education, various lifestyles are often presented on equal levels, and the drawbacks are sometimes downplayed or omitted. This is particularly true regarding cohabitation, which is often presented as a positive experience that enables two people to determine if they are suited for marriage. The assumption is that a "trial marriage" will help to screen out incompatible couples, thereby producing future marriages with greater satisfaction, communication, and commitment. However, studies of cohabitors show that the opposite tends to occur.

In the *Journal of Marriage and the Family*, DeMaris and Leslie investigated 309 recently married couples and found that premarital cohabitation was associated with significantly lower perceived quality of communication for wives and significantly lower marital satisfaction for both spouses. The authors concluded, contrary to their original expectations, that cohabitation does not improve mate selection.

The University of Wisconsin sociologists also showed that cohabitation does not result in better marriages. Of the 13,000 people studied, those who lived together before marriage were twice as likely to get divorced within the first ten years of marriage as those who had not.[146]

Thus, presenting premarital cohabitation as an advantageous lifestyle is contrary to scientific findings.

H. COMPREHENSIVE SEX EDUCATION AND THEORIES OF SEXUAL DEVELOPMENT

Comprehensive sex educators have developed programs for the classroom without regard to the proper age level and sexual development of students. Originally, advocates recommended programs at the secondary level and for the prepuberty years. But now they have pushed for kindergarten through twelfth grade programs and for "comprehensive" coverage of information. Essentially, their agenda permits the full discussion of human sexuality. They believe that children at young ages should be shown explicit illustrations and taught physiological as well as slang terminology for the genitalia and sexual intercourse. They believe young people should be told about alternative lifestyles in a values-neutral context, without reference to marriage and commitment.[147] The Guttmacher Institute labels objections to this approach as complaints by the religious Right.[148]

When Surgeon General Koop called for kindergarten through twelfth grade sex education,[149] many sex educators used the opportunity to justify the above methodology. Considering that two-thirds of school districts in large cities already offer sex education at the elementary level,[150] there seems to be no shortage of such programs. But even the threat of AIDS is not justifiable grounds to expand such programs and to become more explicit. In the U.S., of the 44,395 cases of AIDS reported, only 183 were children. This amounts to just 1 child in every 90 school districts having AIDS.[151] Of those children who have AIDS, 78.1 percent obtained it from an infected mother in utero or during birth, 17.4 percent contracted it from the transfusion of blood or blood components, and 4.4 percent got it from undetermined sources.[152] These statistics show that the AIDS incidence among children is very small, and that those who did contract the disease did not obtain it by being involved in risk-taking behavior.

In terms of sexual development, children from about age six through puberty are in the latency state, during which their sexual energy and thoughts are dormant, and natural inhibitions and repulsion toward sexual topics serve to protect them. But rather than allowing these sexual impulses to remain dormant, sex educators can stir them up through explicitness.[153] And most sex education at the elementary school level is inappropriate in this regard.

The testimonies of experts in child development confirm the dangers of sex education during the latency period. Dr. John Meek, director of child and adolescent services at the Psychiatric Institute of Washington, says, "It is clear that **sexual instruction in the lower elementary grades is unwarranted and potentially destructive to a large percentage of our children**" (emphasis added).[154]

Dr. Sean O'Reilly, professor at the school of medicine and health services at George Washington University, holds the same view:

> Provision of detailed sex instruction either in the co-educational classroom or in private to pre-pubertal children is **ill-advised and potentially harmful.** The professional reason for this fact is the existence and importance of the latency period in human personality growth and development. This is a period of varying duration, in most cases covering the ages of six until puberty, during which thoughts about sexual matters are minimal (emphasis added).

Dr. O'Reilley points out that the consensus of the members of the American Association of Child Psychoanalysis was that **the child's development is not served by encouraging sexuality at this stage of life.**[155]

Dr. Myre Sim, professor of psychiatry at the University of Ottawa, agrees that "it should be recognized that **the school structure and grading system...are unsatisfactory for teaching sex to children.**" She concurs also that disturbances of the latency period interfere with the most productive learning phase in child development and in this respect, it is "anti-educational."[156]

Dr. Rhoda L. Lorand, a psychoanalyst, says that these programs promote "unhealthy sex absorption" and "primitive behavior."[157] These testimonies should lead policy makers to the conclusion expressed by Dr. David Elkind, professor of child study at Tufts University, in his book *The Hurried Child:*

> There is far from total agreement as to whether sex education in the schools is beneficial to **any** age group, much less to young people approaching adolescence. One has to conclude that sex education in the schools reflects adult anxiety about young people's sexuality. The "prejudice" that early sex education will produce children with "healthy sexuality" is open to serious question—even if experts agreed as to what healthy sexuality is—which they do not. Sex education in the schools, given at even younger ages and without clear-cut theoretical or research justification, is another way in which some contemporary schools are encouraging their pupils to grow up fast.[158]

I. COMPREHENSIVE SEX EDUCATION AND THEORIES OF COGNITIVE DEVELOPMENT

Sex education has been shown to be inappropriate for elementary school because it adversely affects the development of children during the latency stage. As if that were not bad enough, once children enter puberty and are subjected to additional sex courses, they then suffer from additional poorly designed programs—namely, those that follow wrong theories of adolescent cognitive development. While the adolescent years are appropriate times for young people to be given guidance regarding sexuality, most sex education courses are designed for adult reasoning rather than adolescent thinking abilities.

Dr. Wanda Franz, associate professor of child development and family studies at West Virginia University, notes that "the courses are failing because they have failed to evaluate the cognitive nature of the adolescent audience that they are attempting to reach. The courses are not designed to accommodate the needs and cognitive limitations of the adolescent population."

Dr. Franz points out four false generalities on which contemporary sex education is based:

Myth #1: Adolescents function like adults and can be expected to make logical decisions.
Myth #2: Given a wide range of choices about sexual lifestyles, the adolescent will choose one rationally.
Myth #3: Teenagers must inevitably engage in sexual behavior.
Myth #4: Adolescents can be taught the meaning of love and will engage in responsible love-making.[159]

To discredit these myths, Franz refers to Piaget's stages of cognitive development, which are listed in Table 13.

Table 13
Piaget's Stages of Cognitive Development

Stage	Age
Sensorimotor	0–2 years
Pre-operational	3–6 years
Concrete operational	7–11 years
Formal operational	*12 years upward

* Research shows that this number has risen to age 18 or over.

While it would appear from Piaget's chart that teens are at the adult reasoning stage, numerous studies show that today's adolescents are still in the concrete, not formal operations, stage. It is rare for an adolescent to function in the formal operations stage.[160]

To illustrate the difference between the concrete and formal operator, Dr. Franz sets up a contrastive chart using Piaget's insights, as seen in Table 14.[161]

Table 14
Concrete Versus Formal Operator

Concrete Operator (adolescent)	Formal Operator (adult)
— Overwhelmed by immediate concrete experience	— Anticipates possible outcomes
	— Tests systematically
— Cannot anticipate future outcome	— Considers complex interactions
— Processes in a haphazard way	— Associates behavior with outcome

Adapted from Wanda Franz, "Adolescent Cognitive Abilities and Implications for Sexual Decision-Making." Used with permission of the author.

Given the difference between the concrete and formal operator, it is apparent that the neutral decision-making approach in secondary education is doomed to fail, because it is useful only for adults.

Dr. Franz further pursues the subject of cognitive development specifically as it pertains to decisions regarding sexual activity. Again using a contrastive chart (see Table 15), Franz shows the differences between the concrete and formal operator, clearly suggesting that neutral decision-making models for adolescents are particularly inappropriate as they pertain to sexual decision making.[162]

Table 15
Cognitive Development and Decisions About Sexual Activity

Concrete Operator (adolescent)	Formal Operator (adult)
— Immediate sexual gratification	— Considers future risks
— Future risks disregarded	— Recognizes the significance of all possible risks
— Options not evaluated	— Recognizes that sexual activity entails responsibility
— Responsibility for actions not evaluated	

Adapted from Wanda Franz, "Adolescent Cognitive Abilities and Implications for Sexual Decision-Making." Used with permission of the author.

Franz then carries the chart one step further and applies it to love, showing that the concrete operator is incapable of true love, whereas the formal operator can participate in genuine love, as seen in Table 16.[163]

Table 16
Cognitive Development as It Pertains to Love

Concrete Operator (adolescent)	Formal Operator (adult)
— Immediate sexual gratification	— Sex for love and procreation
— Self-indulgence	— Concern for partner
— Self-knowledge	— Self-giving
— Short-term relationships	— Long-term commitment

Adapted from Wanda Franz, "Adolescent Cognitive Abilities and Implications for Sexual Decision-Making." Used with permission of the author.

Thus, on the basis of current theories of cognitive development, it is apparent that adolescents cannot be expected to make logical decisions or use formal operational thought regarding sexual activity; that given a wide range of choices, they will not choose one rationally; and that they cannot be expected to understand and participate in true love. (See also the findings of Jorgensen in section IV.A.) These realities should help decision makers in the schools understand that the values-neutral decision-making models in comprehensive sex education are inappropriate.

J. COMPREHENSIVE SEX EDUCATION AND THEORIES OF ETHICAL DEVELOPMENT

Dr. Franz has shown not only that comprehensive sex education goes contrary to adolescent cognitive development, but that it is also inappropriate relative to the state of adolescent moral development. To prove her point, Franz cites Kohlberg's stages of moral reasoning,[164] listed in Table 17.

Table 17
Kohlberg's Stages of Moral Reasoning

1. **Might makes right:** fear of punishment controls action.

2. **Hedonism:** opportunity for pleasure controls action.

3. **Social acceptance:** value by respected others controls action.

4. **Role of law:** following the rule controls action.

5. **Contractual:** human responsibilities control action.

6. **Principled:** system of higher principles controls action.

Adapted from Wanda Franz "Adolescent Cognitive Abilities and the Implications for Sexual Decision-Making." Used with permission of the author.

Today's adolescents rarely function above the fourth of Kohlberg's stages.[165] Therefore, whenever they make decisions, they are relying not on logical reasoning but on the first four stages of moral reasoning.

On the negative side of moral reasoning, the first stage, "Might makes right," accounts for "date rape." But on the positive side, the fear of punishment from parents, God, or law enforcers (as in the case of rape) will cause young people to abstain.

The second stage, "hedonism," accounts for indulgence in sexual gratification. Unfortunately, our society is filled with messages from the media, music, and even certain laws (e.g. abortion on demand) that encourage teens to engage in sex in a hedonistic way without acknowledging consequences.

In a negative way, the third stage of "social acceptance" causes teens to give in to sex because "everyone is doing it" and it is socially acceptable. And when sex educators say to teens in a classroom setting, "We know you're involved in sex," "This is normal behavior," and "Use contraceptives if you are going to be sexually active," teens will have increased support for the view that sexual intercourse among adolescents is socially acceptable. But when parents, educators, peers, clergy, and respected others indicate that premarital sexual intercourse is unacceptable, many teens will be positively influenced to abstain.

Stage four, "role of law," is built upon the earlier stages, and when laws are verbalized to teens, they can know if they are obeying. Rules can come from peers, parents, schools, clergy, government, and other sources. Unfortunately, in values-neutral sex education, students are not given the laws of right and wrong. Instead, relativistic values clarification is used.[166]

Secretary of Education William Bennett, who served during a time when sex education became a national issue, criticized sex education for taking a neutral stance on rules. He observed:

Indeed, you sometimes get the feeling that, for these guides, being "comfortable" with one's decision when exercising one's "option" is the sum and substance of the responsible life. Decisions aren't right or wrong—decisions simply make you comfortable or not. It is as though "comfort" alone had now become our moral compass.[167]

Comprehensive sex educators often say they cannot teach morals in the classroom because "morals are so subjective" and "whose morals are we going to teach, anyway?" Yet, the cultural norm in the United States still favors premarital abstinence and shows disfavor toward casual sex among minors. Nevertheless, progressive sex educators believe they need to avoid upholding normative standards. And because of the inappropriate, adult decision-making models used in the classroom, adolescents have no recourse but to make their sexual decisions on the basis of the first four stages of moral reasoning. Therefore, when comprehensive educators list "value neutrality" as an asset to their programs, they are unknowingly acknowledging a major flaw. School personnel examining various sex education programs would be wise to avoid values-neutral programs and look for materials designed to communicate with the adolescent mode of thinking.

In view of these findings, schools should carefully examine their existing sex education programs, remove questionable materials, and avoid approaches that will not only fail to solve the adolescent sexuality crisis, but also produce harmful consequences for the young people they are trying to help.

William Bennett accurately sums up the approach of contemporary sex education:

> What's wrong with this kind of teaching? First, it is a very odd kind of teaching—very odd because it does not teach. It does not teach because, while speaking to a very important aspect of human life, it displays a conscious aversion to making moral distinctions.... What is being done in these classes is tantamount to throwing up our hands and saying to our young people, "We give up. We give up. We give up on teaching right and wrong to you. Here, take these facts, take this information, and take your feelings, your options, and try to make the best decisions you can. But you're on your own. We can say no more."[168]

IV. *INFLUENCING TODAY'S YOUTH*

An adolescent sexuality crisis exists in the United States, one that was virtually nonexistent a few decades ago, and one that could continue to worsen. When pondering how to intervene, the minority members of the U. S. House Select Committee on Children, Youth, and Families questioned:

Every generation has inherited the difficult job of bringing children into adulthood, and the same problems have presented themselves. Why is it so different now? Why does the problem seem so much more difficult in this generation? Are babies born today different from babies born fifty years ago? Or is the difference in the adults raising them?[169]

Table 18
Estimated Shifts in the Influences Upon 13- to 19-year-olds
Who Change Their Values and Behavior

1960	1980	
1st mother, father	1st friends, peers	(UP 2)
2nd teachers	2nd mother, father	(DOWN 1)
3rd friends, peers	3rd television, radio, records, cinema	(UP 5)
4th ministers, priests, rabbis	4th teachers	(DOWN 2)
5th youth club leaders, counselors, advisers, Scoutmasters, coaches, librarians	5th popular heroes, idols in sports, music	(UP 1)
6th popular heroes, idols in sports, music	6th ministers, priests, rabbis	(DOWN 2)
7th grandparents, uncles, aunts	7th newspapers, magazines	(UP 2)
8th television, records, cinema, radio	8th advertising	(UP 2)
9th magazines, newspapers	9th youth club leaders, counselors, advisers, Scoutmasters, coaches, librarians	(DOWN 4)
10th advertising	10th grandparents, uncles, aunts	(DOWN 3)

Johnston Company synthesis of 18 studies for youth and values-oriented clients, 1954–80, as listed in McDowell's Research Digest. *Used with the permission of Josh McDowell Ministries.*

A. NEGATIVE INFLUENCES AND BARRIERS TO REACHING YOUTH

Adults who want to reach adolescents need to realize that a major shift has taken place in American culture regarding the influences on today's youth. Between 1960 and 1980, parents, teachers, school officials and club leaders, clergy, and relatives **all dropped in their level of influence over youth.** Friends and peers, on the other hand, have become far more influential, as have television, radio, records, movies, popular heroes, sports and music idols, newspapers, magazines, and advertising. Table 18 lists the various shifts in influences upon teens during the twenty-year span.[170]

The net result of these shifts in influence on teens is seen most dramatically in the detrimental sexual consequences. The summary chart in Table 19 reveals the trends in conception among females ages fifteen to nineteen during the relatively short time span of five years.[171]

Table 19
Trends in Conception Among Women 15–19 Years of Age

Item	1974	1979	Percentage Change
1. Women 15–19	10,186,000	10,145,000	—
2. Birth rate (per 1000)	58.7	53.4	– 9.0
3. Sexual activity Ever married	1,272,000	894,000	– 29.7
Never married women who are sexually active	2,888,000	3,922,000	+ 35.8
Percentage never married who are sexually active	32.4	42.4	+ 30.9
4. Women at risk of pregnancy (ever married and sexually active never married)	4,160,000	4,816,000	+ 15.8
5. Births	594,400	549,500	– 7.6
6. Births per 1000 sexually active	143.1	114.1	– 20.3
7. Induced abortions	278,300	449,500	+ 61.5
8. Estimated conceptions (births and induced abortions)	873,700	999,000	+ 14.3
9. Conceptions per 1000 women	85.8	98.5	+ 14.8
10. Conceptions per 1000 sexually active women	210.0	207.4	– 1.2
11. Abortions per 1000 sexually active women	66.9	93.9	+ 39.5

(Adapted from Baldwin, W: Adolescent Pregnancy and Childbearing—Growing Concerns for Americans. Popul. Bull. 31:1–36, 1980, updated reprint.) As listed in McDowell's Research Digest. Used with the permission of Josh McDowell Ministries.

After 1979, the pregnancy rate for women age fifteen to nineteen climbed still higher, going to 111 per 1,000 women in 1980 and still at 108 per 1,000 in 1983. The live birth rate actually declined slightly in this age group, from 53 per 1,000 in 1980 to 50.9 in 1984. The number of abortions continued to increase.

Overcoming the negative influences and reversing the trends is a difficult task. During the past twenty years, the contraceptive approach in family planning services, school-based clinics, and comprehensive sex education has failed. Researchers Olsen, Wallace, and Miller have accurately pinpointed the reason for this failure, saying that "it isolates the causes of adolescent pregnancy and its symptoms from the contexts in which they occur." They give this description of what the broad picture should properly entail:

> The larger context consists of the family of the adolescent and attending family values; the adolescent peer group and values; the thinking processes and reasoning skills of the parents and adolescents; and the values and behavior of the adolescent couple involved in sexual activity. The reason these areas are addressed is that teenage sexual decision making has implications for teens, for their families, and for society. These consequences are not just physical and economic, but also social and emotional, immediate as well as long-term.[172]

While there need to be several community sources that address these contexts, the school system is an appropriate setting in which parents and teachers can work together. Obviously, the task is not easy, and there are many obstacles that reduce effectiveness. Olson, Wallace, and Miller[173] refer to the research of Jorgensen, who identified four contextual barriers to reducing adolescent pregnancies by educational means:

1. *There are those teenage girls who intentionally become pregnant to escape family conflict.* The desire to have a baby who will presumably give and receive love is a strong temptation to an adolescent girl who foresees no change in her troubled home life.

   Zelnik and Kantner report that about 28 percent of teen pregnancies are intended,[174] a view substantiated by Dr. Harriet McAdoo[175] and reporter Leon Dash.[176]

2. *The stage of adolescent cognitive development contributes to immature sexual decision making.* As stated earlier in this report (see section III), Dr. Wanda Franz's analysis of adolescent cognitive abilities shows that teens do not make long-range, adult-like decisions about sex and its consequences.

3. *Sex-role structures in today's society encourage a noncommitted, promiscuous lifestyle for teens.* Hedonism then becomes a basis on which adolescents make moral decisions (See section III.).

4. *There is inadequate parental involvement in educating children about sexuality.*

B. OVERCOMING THE BARRIERS TO REACHING TODAY'S YOUTH

While the four obstacles to reducing teenage pregnancy may seem insurmountable, Olson, Wallace, and Miller propose that the barriers become a focal point around which to build a primary prevention program, one that targets the entire adolescent population while also building on the family context.[177]

1. *Overcoming intentional pregnancies that occur as a result of a poor home life.* Olson, Wallace, and Miller acknowledge that the nearly one-third of pregnancies that are intentional are the most formidable obstacle to overcome, and that if family problems are the contributing factor, the likelihood of positive parental involvement in sex education is remote. The researchers recommend other means to attack this barrier:

    A. Teach adolescents alternative ways of coping with family conflict besides becoming pregnant. Conflict resolution techniques can be introduced. Other means of achieving a sense of belonging can be explored.

    B. Teach long-range effects of adolescent pregnancy for the adolescent, the infant, and the family.

    C. Help to improve the quality of family life for the high-risk teen.

    Counselors who interact with adolescent girls in this high-risk category confirm that this type of intervention is vital.[178]

2. *Overcoming immature adolescent reasoning.* Olson, Wallace, and Miller propose tangible ways to help develop more mature adolescent reasoning by educational means:[179]

    A. Exclude children from fully exercising their choices. The reason the American democratic system protects adolescents is that it recognizes they are not adults. The system is designed to help youth move toward mature moral development and reasoning that will eventually grant them full entitlement of democratic rights. Until then, teens are protected by adults and the system, and they are not held accountable for adult behavior.

    B. Show that hedonistic philosophies undermine responsible decision making.

    C. Teach negotiation skills that would serve in the best interest of all involved.

    D. Help adolescents to ponder questions about the meaning of justice and integrity and to develop criteria for doing so. Help them to transfer these criteria to various contexts, including educational, financial, and relational situations.

    E. Do not allow discussion to be conducted objectively, with every option considered equal in weight. Include moral implications for all choices.

    F. Do not allow "voting" to determine what is right and wrong.

    G. Prepare take-home activities so that insights from classroom discussion can be overseen by parents, who will then add a sense of permanence, authority, and love to the value system being developed in the adolescent.

3. *Overcoming the permissive norms established in emotionally intimate adolescent couples.* Olson, Wallace, and Miller point out that most adolescent couples live in a fantasy and do not have a mature sense of justice, responsibility, and honesty.[180] To overcome this barrier, they propose the following:

    A. Focus on cognitive development as discussed in overcoming barrier number 2.

    B. Explore the different motivations and meanings for male and female sexual involvement.

    C. Show how the consequences of premarital sex weigh most heavily on females, but that both the male and female may suffer. Mention paternity laws.

4. *Overcoming the lack of parental involvement in the education of children about sexuality.* Olson, Wallace, and Miller show that lack of knowledge about biological facts or parental values may not be a major contributing factor in teen pregnancies.[181] Instead, the conflict between teen behavior and parental values tends to be the typical scenario.

Conflicts between teen behavior and parental values can be explored as linesof communication are opened by teaching moral reasoning skills to parents and teens, enabling them to address common issues. When teens are able to side with parental values, they are more likely to abstain from sexual intercourse. Section VI. of this report will discuss the ways in which parental involvement is being enhanced through programs in the schools.

C. OTHER FACTORS CORRELATED WITH APPROPRIATE ADOLESCENT SEXUAL BEHAVIOR

There are other factors that positively influence adolescent sexual behavior of which parents and educators need to be aware. The first eight factors are cited as test results of the AANCHOR curriculum.[182]

Table 20
Percentage of Never-Married Teenagers Having Had
Sexual Intercourse, Based on Parental Strictness, 1983

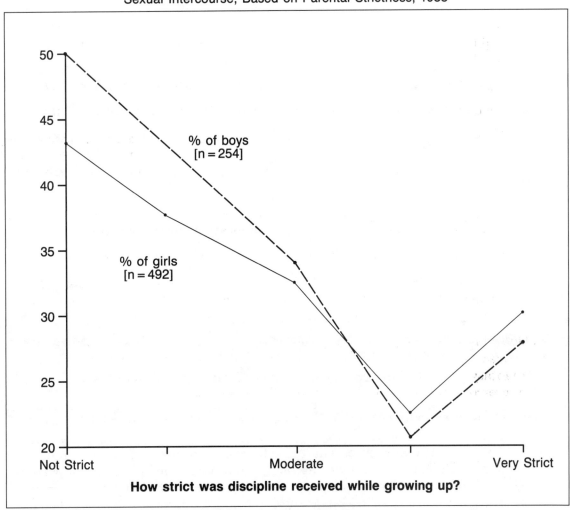

From Olson and Wallace, A Sampler of AANCHOR. *Used with permission.*

1. A strong personal belief that premarital intercourse is usually or always wrong is a contributor to adolescent virginity.

2. Adolescents living with both parents have the least permissive views of premarital sex, followed by those living with a parent who has remarried.

3. Teenagers who report their parents' discipline to be "moderately high" are twice as likely as those whose parents are "not strict at all" to avoid premarital intercourse, as seen in Table 20.[183]

4. Teens who report that their parents have moderately strict rules about dating are more likely to abstain than those who have no rules or excessive rules,[184] as seen in Table 21.

Table 21
Percentage of Never-Married Teenagers Having Had Sexual Intercourse,
Based on Number of Parental Dating Rules, 1983

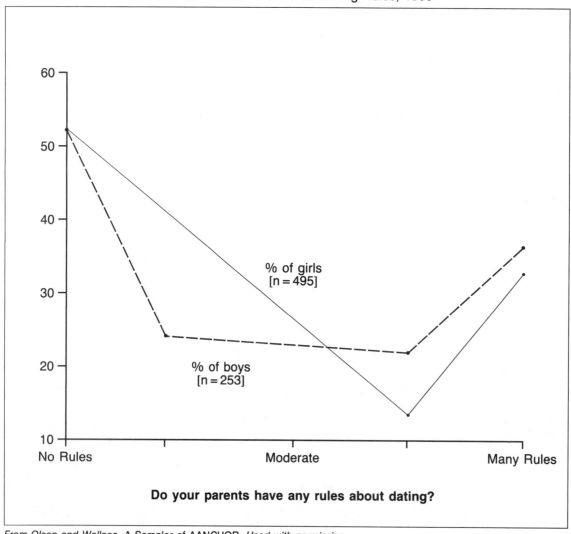

From Olson and Wallace, A Sampler of AANCHOR. *Used with permission.*

5. Teens who report that their parents are interested and involved in their grades and personal achievements are twice as likely to abstain from sex as those who say their parents do not feel their grades or achievements are important.

6. Teens who attain high academic grades are more likely to abstain.

7. Teens who look to the future by making plans for higher education are more likely to abstain than those who don't.

8. Teens who delay starting to date and avoid steady dating are more likely to abstain, as shown in Table 22.[185]

Table 22
Percentage of Teenage Girls Having Had Sexual Intercourse.
Based on the Age Dating Began

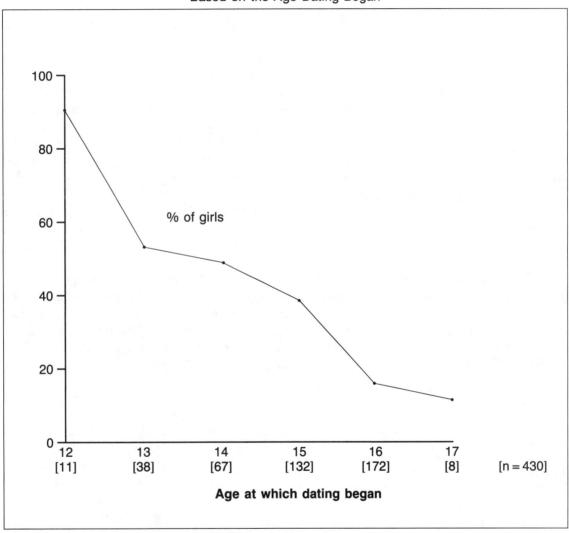

9. Teens who report that religion is important to them are more likely to abstain.

10. Teenage girls who report a close mother-daughter relationship are more likely to abstain.[186]

D. PERCENTAGE RATES OF VIRGINS AND SECONDARY VIRGINS

Given the studies showing there are tangible ways to reach adolescents and that there are positive influences on teens to abstain from sex, educators and parents can take hope. Even more encouraging are the statistics showing that not all teens are sexually active.

Zelnik and Kantner indicated that the majority of high school students in the 1970s were virgins.[187] Even in the 1980s, the statistics hold true. Studies from 1981, 1983, 1986, and 1987 show that about half of all eighteen-year-olds have never had premarital intercourse.[188] Moreover, the percentage of black youths who are sexually active is on the decline. Considering the high percentage of teens who are abstaining, educators **must** implement programs that will protect, not harm, these students.

In spite of the statistics showing the high percentage of teens who are virgins, there is a prevailing misconception that "everyone is doing it." A Louis Harris poll showed that 90 percent of teens admitted they had become promiscuous simply because of **perceived** peer pressure. Of those who had had sex, 80 percent said they felt they had been drawn into sex too soon.[189] Regret often causes such teens to cut back on sexual behavior; unfortunately, teens who have had sex only once are classified as "sexually active," inflating the teenage promiscuity rate.

Researchers Zelnik and Kantner, who interviewed teens who have had sex, found that only half had had intercourse during the month prior to their interview. Half the "sexually active" girls had had only one partner, and 14 percent had had intercourse only once.[190]

Regarding the relative inactivity and return to abstinence among teens who had had sexual intercourse, it is realistic to promote "secondary virginity." As Dr. James Ford notes, "These figures indicate that secondary virginity is not all that rare among teenagers. In other words, an appreciable percentage of unmarried teenagers who have experienced premarital intercourse are not currently 'sexually active.'"[191] The numbers of teens who are truly sexually active are relatively few.

V. ABSTINENCE EDUCATION

For more than two thousand years, Western civilization believed in premarital abstinence and accepted it as a cultural norm. Human sexuality was channeled away from self-indulgence and toward fruitful ends. While it was not a perfect system, it acted as the greatest deterrent to out-of-wedlock pregnancies.[192]

The past two decades have been different, however. Relaxed standards have permitted adolescents to engage in premarital intercourse, accompanied by the blessings of family planning advocates who have offered a pill or an abortion to resolve unwanted pregnancies. But now there is a clear movement underway that rebuffs the laxity in morality and upholds high standards for teenagers. Dr. David Schaff, a psychoanalyst, observes: "The whole culture is on a swing back to more traditional expectations. There is a return to the understanding that the main function of sex is the bodily expression of intimacy."[193]

A. THE ABSTINENCE MOVEMENT

In the *Medical World News,* Alexandra Mark, Ph.D., and Vernon H. Mark, M.D., challenge leaders across the nation to take a stand regarding abstinence:

> The mounting evidence indicting the leaders of the sexual revolution is impressive. They promised joy, liberation, and good health. They've delivered misery, disease, and even death.... The answer is that we must recognize that the appeal for a change to responsible behavior has to start at the top levels...[groups] that now must discard [their] apathy, get involved, and present the young with a better vision of the future, consistent with sexual responsibility.[194]

1. Federal Legislation

The greatest support for abstinence education came from the federal government. In 1981, President Ronald Reagan signed into law the Adolescent Family Life Act of Title XX of the Public Health Service Act. The law is administered by the Office of Adolescent Pregnancy Programs within the Office of Population Affairs of the Department of Health and Human Services. Among the unique features of the Adolescent Family Life Act is its emphasis on the importance of family involvement; the promotion of adolescent premarital sexual abstinence; good parenting; adoption; and comprehensive health, education, and social services to help an expectant teenager have a healthy baby. The total number of projects funded since the onset has been ninety-seven. Currently, the program is funding twenty-eight prevention programs promoting parental involvement and abstinence.[195] The effectiveness of some of these programs is discussed in Section V. G. of this report.

2. National Government Experts

National government leaders have also endorsed morally based abstinence education. President Reagan said, "To teach sex as a purely physical function without taking into consideration the moral precepts that are involved—I think that should be of concern to those in charge of education." In September 1988, he also directed the Secretary of Health and Human Services to ensure that all "human sexuality and family planning educational and informational materials developed for teens by Federal agencies and, to the extent permitted by law, grantees focus on promoting and encouraging abstinence." And he ordered the secretary to propose legislation or take administrative action so that federal funds would not be used to distribute "contraceptives or prescriptions for contraceptives in schools without parental permission."[196]

Gary Bauer, who served as undersecretary of education before becoming President Reagan's aide on policy development, underscored the same point, saying, "Most responsible parents have instinctively known that adult leadership in any sex education program must provide a moral foundation, without which instability is permanently nailed to our children's future."[197]

Said William Bennett:

Sex education has to do with how boys and girls, how men and women should treat each other and themselves. Sex education is therefore about character and the formation of character. A sex education course in which issues of right and wrong do not occupy center stage is an evasion and an irresponsibility.[198]

In a joint statement with Surgeon General Koop, Bennett also said:

Young people must be told the truth—that the best way to avoid AIDS is to refrain from sexual activity, until, as adults, they are ready to establish a mutually faithful, monogamous relationship. Since sex education courses should in any case teach children why they should refrain from engaging in sexual intercourse, AIDS (as part of sex education in general) should uphold monogamy in marriage as a desirable and worthy thing.[199]

JoAnn Gasper, former deputy assistant secretary for population affairs of the Department of Health and Human Services and a former aide to William Bennett in the Department of Education, also upholds the importance of abstinence education, pointing out that "sexual abstinence is the only foolproof way of not getting pregnant. The message to convey is you do not engage in sex until marriage."[200]

3. Medical Associations

Some medical associations have also issued resolutions favoring adolescent abstinence. In 1984, the California Medical Association passed a statement eventually adopted by the American Medical Association that same year:

Unwanted pregnancy, especially among teenagers, is a serious problem, and [since] it is appropriate for CMA to support, through health education activities, teenagers who wish to resist peer pressure to engage in premarital sexual activities; now therefore, be it resolved that CMA recognizes that premarital abstinence is an effective means of precluding unwanted pregnancy; and be it further resolved that CMA suggests that the media, appropriate public agencies, and all concerned professional groups, in their educational campaigns to the public, emphasize the effectiveness of premarital abstinence as a means of reducing the incidence of unwanted pregnancy.[201]

An adolescent abstinence resolution was also passed at the September 1987 meeting of the Chapter Forum of the American Academy of Pediatrics (AAP). Final wording and approval of the resolution is pending review by the adolescent committee and the executive board of the AAP. The version passed at the Chapter Forum reads as follows:

Whereas over one million teenage girls become pregnant each year, and Whereas the incidence of sexually transmitted disease in the adolescent population remains a major health concern, Herpes and AIDS currently have no cure and venereal warts are recognized as carcinogenic viruses, and Whereas teen use of contraceptives has been shown to be unreliable, and Whereas abortion, with its immediate and long-range health consequences, is a poor method of birth control, and Whereas the AAP should set an example for media, public agencies, and concerned professional groups,

Be it resolved, that the AAP recommends that adolescents postpone, until marriage, sexual activities that may lead to pregnancy or sexually transmitted diseases.[202]

4. State Legislators

While many states have for years required that sex education be taught in the public schools, some states are now recognizing that abstinence must serve as the underlying perspective in such programs. Illinois became the leading state to pass an abstinence education bill.[203] Indiana also legislated abstinence education by passing two bills. One pertains to AIDS education and went into effect on January 1, 1988.[204] The other covers several educational areas and became effective July 1, 1988.

In March 1988, the state of Washington passed the AIDS Omnibus Bill requiring AIDS education in all public schools, with an emphasis on premarital abstinence as the only sure way to avoid contracting the disease sexually.[205] In Florida, an AIDS legislative package also upheld the teaching of abstinence and emphasized it as the expected norm for adolescents.[206]

In August 1988, California also passed an abstinence education bill. It, too, calls for promoting abstinence as the only certain way to avoid pregnancy, sexually transmitted diseases, and the sexual transmission of AIDS. It further requires that monogamous heterosexual marriage be treated with honor and respect in all materials and instruction.[207]

In April 1988, Kentucky Governor Wilkinson signed into law a parental education and family life skills act that has, as one of its provisions, an emphasis on premarital abstinence.[208]

In December 1987, the Missouri Task Force on Unwed Adolescent Sexual Activity and Pregnancy, authorized by the state, issued the report, *A Time to Speak. . . A Time to Act*. In the opening statements of the report, Jerome Shen, M.D., chairman of the task force, said:

> With faith and optimism, the Task Force is confident that the goal of deterring unwed adolescent sexual activity and pregnancy can be achieved if we attack basic causes and eliminate long-tried yet unsuccessful programs; emphasize individual, family, and societal morals; encourage chastity, parental authority, responsibility, and family communication; respect for children's rights and promote innovative programs.[209]

In just the first few months of 1989, many abstinence education bills have been introduced and are under current review, suggesting that policy-makers across the country are exploring this approach. Among those states are Arizona, Florida, Montana, New Jersey, Oklahoma, and Texas.[210]

Several other states have recently rejected proposed legislation that would have mandated kindergarten through twelfth grade comprehensive sex education not taughtfrom the perspective of premarital abstinence. Among them are Pennsylvania, Texas, and Louisiana.[211]

5. School Officials

While some states have chosen to mandate the teaching of abstinence by passing legislation, other states have chosen to require abstinence education as a result of efforts on the part of their state board of education. In January 1988, the New York State Board of Regents mailed to all (over 700) its school districts the third revision of its manual on AIDS education. Formerly, the manual stressed condoms and "safe sex," but the new manual emphasizes abstinence as the only sure way to avoid AIDS.

The change in the New York manual is credited to the efforts of the Grand Island School District, an area near Buffalo. The Grand Island school board members alerted the State Board of the inappropriateness of most AIDS educational materials, and their decision to endorse abstinence education. Throughout the state of New York, school districts have turned to Grand Island for help. The State Board of Regents not only adopted the advice of Grand Island, but it instructed local school districts to set up advisory councils in order to assure that programs would be acceptable to community standards. [212]

Many public school districts are coming to the conclusion that past programs need to be abandoned in favor of new approaches. When school officials in San Marcos, California, discovered that one in five high school girls had become pregnant one year, they decided to take action. As Joe DeDiminicantanio, principal at San Marcos Junior High, describes:

> A quick, knee-jerk reaction to the problem about teenage pregnancies would have been to have hauled all of the girls in the gym and all of the boys in another gym and shown them some movies and told them where to buy prophylactics. But what we really want to do is change behaviors and influence attitudes, and that will take some time.[213]

San Marcos school officials adopted an abstinence program from Teen-Aid and developed their own in-house esteem-building program. (Section V.G.3. of this report discusses the results.)

In addition to school superintendents and principals, teachers are also expressing favor for abstinence programs. In describing the *Sex Respect* curricula, one teacher expressed a view held by many, saying that in the past, teachers "felt like what we were doing really wasn't the answer."[214]

In some school districts, school boards and parents are working together for the implementation of an abstinence policy. Northside Independent School District in suburban San Antonio adopted a policy which includes support for sexual abstinence before marriage, limits contraceptive education only to those students whose parents specifically request it, and requires the age and maturity of students to be considered in the selection of instructional materials.

6. The Media

Endorsements of abstinence education are also coming from the national media. Some reporters and columnists are beginning to step forward and take a stand for morality. Dr. Art Ulene, family physician to NBC's "Today Show," said in June 1987: "I think it's time to stop talking about 'safe sex'. . . . I believe that complete abstention from sexual activities with others is a choice that deserves serious consideration in the age of AIDS. . . . I believe that abstinence is an especially good option for the youngsters of our world."[215]

Ted Koppel, ABC's "Nightline" host, emphasized sexual morality in a speech he gave at Duke University in 1987:

> We have actually convinced ourselves that slogans will save us. "Shoot up if you must, but use a clean needle." "Enjoy sex whenever and with whomever you wish, but wear a condom." No! That answer is no. Not because it isn't cool or smart or because you might end up in jail or dying in an AIDS ward, but no because it's wrong, because we have spent 5,000 years as a race of rational human beings, trying to drag ourselves out of the primeval slime by searching for truth and moral absolutes. In its purest form, truth is not a polite tap on the shoulder. It is a howling reproach. What Moses brought down from Mount Sinai were not the Ten Suggestions.[216]

Syndicated columnist William Raspberry has written several columns calling for young people to abstain from sex and for schools to teach morality. In support of former Secretary of Education William Bennett, Raspberry says:

> Are we ready to make a similar assumption when it comes to sexual activity among teenagers? Are we prepared to concede that they will do things we know are not in their best interest? Well, some of us will insist, with Bennett. . ., that when it comes to sex, the only acceptable instruction adults can offer adolescents is "Don't."[217]

B. MYTHS ABOUT ABSTINENCE EDUCATION

School officials often have some skepticism about abstinence education. When the facts are clarified, however, schools can feel comfortable with the approach.

1. Is Abstinence Education Religious Indoctrination?

Perhaps the greatest misunderstanding about abstinence education is the belief that it is religious in nature, and therefore it violates the Establishment Clause of the U.S. Constitution. Opponents are saying that because abstinence is the conduct upheld in the Bible, as well as in the works of some of the other major world religions, it is exclusively a religious perspective. However, abstinence is also a medical, psychological, sociological, and moral issue. It is on these bases that abstinence can be presented in the public schools.

Another way to see the fallacy of the "religious" argument is to realize that schools already teach it is wrong to steal, cheat, lie, rape, murder, get drunk, and other acts that are harmful to both the individual and others. Schools also teach the positive attributes of charity, love, gratitude, forgiveness, and other favorable traits. These issues, too, are addressed in world religions, but school officials do not consider them to be in conflict with the mission of schools.

Nevertheless, it took the U. S. Supreme Court to finally resolve the dispute, coming down in favor of abstinence education, saying that it can be taught in public schools and that it is not a violation of the Establishment Clause.

On June 29, 1988, the U. S. Supreme Court delivered an opinion in the case of Bowen v. Kendrick. The decision upheld the constitutionality of the Adolescent Family Life Act of 1981 (AFLA), which provides funds for adolescent pregnancy care services and adolescent abstinence education programs. The AFLA states that federally provided services in this area should involve parents and should "emphasize the provision of support by other family members, religious and charitable organizations, voluntary associations, and other groups." Some of the groups that receive the grants are affiliated with churches. The Court upheld the rights of these groups to receive the grants and ruled that it did not violate the Establishment Clause of the first amendment. This means that even when a religious organization goes into the public schools to give presentations about the merits of abstinence, the message is not inherently religious, and therefore it has a place in helping to prevent teenage pregnancy. Specifically, the Court stated:

> The facially neutral projects authorized by the AFLA—including pregnancy testing, adoption counseling and referral services, prenatal and postnatal care, educational services, residential care, child care, consumer education, etc.—are not themselves "specifically religious activities," and they are not converted into such activities by the fact that they are carried out by organizations with religious affiliations.[218]

2. Can Morality Be Taught in Schools?

Similar to the myth about abstinence being a religious issue is the belief that morality cannot be taught in public schools. The underlying premise of this view is that the educational environment must operate in a moral vacuum. Teachers can only present various options, the advantages and disadvantages of each, and then leave the final choice to students. This is the prevailing form of decision-making taught in progressive sex education. However, it is **not** the approach used in drug education, driver's education, health education, and other subjects. Whether they realize it or not, schools include a moral basis in all subjects.

As has been discussed earlier in this report (Sections III.H., III.I., as well as V.A.), teenagers need moral guidance because they lack adequate cognitive development to make logical choices. When given only value-neutral decision-making models, teens will make their decisions based on immature moral reasoning, which is often hedonistic in nature. Therefore, schools must include morality in sex education.

3. Is Abstinence Education Idealistic?

Some people believe abstinence is an ideal that was attainable in past generations but not today. The major underlying assumption of this view is that "most kids are doing it." But as has been shown (Section IV.D.), half the teenagers today are virgins, and many more are secondary virgins who have returned to abstinence. Only a relatively small percentage are truly sexually active. Given the number of virgins and secondary virgins, abstinence education is suited for the majority of adolescents.

Apart from the percentages, abstinence education is pragmatic because it is the only approach that offers a foolproof solution to the prevention of teenage pregnancy, sexually transmitted diseases, and the psychological problems that accompany adolescent sexual activity. Section V of this report will show that abstinence education is also pragmatic because it is proving effective in public schools.

4. Is Abstinence Education Designed to Reach Only Middle Class Youths?

Some critics of abstinence education contend that it will not appeal to inner city, minority youths. Basically, what this view implies is that minorities cannot relate to the values of family and marriage, cannot restrain their sexual drives, and have no long-range goals.

While inner city youths are often the victims of broken marriages and destabilized families, it is the responsibility of society, including the schools, to help build a foundation on which adolescents can begin to understand the importance of family and marriage. Of all social groups, those in the inner city are most in need of programs designed to build self-esteem, a sense of responsibility, and an appreciation for a strong, traditional family unit.

The belief that inner city, minority youths cannot restrain themselves in the area of sexuality is unfounded, as well. In fact, the sexual activity rate among unmarried blacks has steadily declined, and the virginity rate has increased.[219]

The Adolescent Family Life Act has funded projects that are specially designed for urban areas. Under such a grant, for example, Atlanta's Grady Memorial Hospital, along with Emory University, developed and tested a program and found that nine out of ten youths want help in saying no to sexual pressure,[220] and that the skill-building techniques of "saying no" help teens postpone sexual activity.[221]

Another successful program reaching high-risk adolescents is the School/Community Program for Sexual Risk Reduction Among Teens, which operated under a federal grant from October 1982 to September 1987 in South Carolina. The program helped reduce the teenage pregnancy rate from 60 per 1,000 females to 25 per 1,000 females.[222]

The notion that inner city parents are not concerned about the sex education of their children is also untrue. For example, when school-based clinics were set up in a minority community in Chicago, there was a strong outcry from neighborhood parents, clergy, and leaders who protested that the contraceptive approach violated their value system. The adults formed a pro-family coalition that is fighting for the restoration of traditional values in the schools.[223]

5. Is Abstinence Education an Attempt to Govern Morality?

Some opponents of abstinence education contend that the teaching of abstinence is an attempt to govern morality, and that there will be those adolescents who will have sex regardless of the number of programs offered in schools. Obviously, the second half of the statement is true. In fact, over the past two thousand years in which premarital abstinence was the cultural norm, there were instances in which teens would have sex and in which the acts would culminate in illegitimate births. Nevertheless, most of society benefited from the standard of premarital abstinence. But as Kurt Back, psychologist at Duke University, argues, assumed difficulties should not stop us from trying to solve the problem:

> In the same way, one might argue that the elimination of racism and sexism could not be effected by changes in social norms. After all, should one interfere in bigotry between consenting adults? The difference in these cases seems to be more a question of where one wants to interfere than where one could. . . . If the problem of teenage pregnancy is serious, one should consider scientific evidence as well as values and knowledge of the justifications and consequences of self-imposed restraint.[224]

6. Do Teenagers Want to Be Taught About Abstinence?

Many people assume teenagers do not consider premarital relations to be a problem and are not interested in values. But even if this were true, it would not justify omitting abstinence education; schools have the responsibility of setting the agenda, not students. Nevertheless, the statement about lack of interest by teenagers is simply untrue.

A national survey found that among all the items teenagers consider to be a problem, premarital relations ranked number one, even higher than teenage pregnancy, as seen in Table 23.[225]

Table 23
Items Teenagers Consider to Be a Problem

Rank	Problem	%
1	premarital relations	99%
2	drug abuse	85%
3	alcoholism	71%
4	suicide	67%
5	teenage pregnancy	44%
6	teen porn & prostitution	15%

As listed in McDowell's Research Digest. *Used with permission of Josh McDowell Ministries.*

In a 1987 survey of teens listed in *Who's Who Among American High School Students,* 59 percent of females and 47 percent of males believed that a discussion of values and morals in sex education would be worthwhile.[226]

Not only are today's adolescents concerned about the morality of premarital sex, but they also want help to resist pressure to be sexually active. As mentioned earlier, Atlanta's Grady Memorial Hospital found that nine out of ten girls interviewed wanted to learn how to say no to sexual pressure.[227]

Eunice Kennedy Shriver, sister of the late president and director of the Kennedy Foundation, has discovered during her twenty-five years as a social worker that teenagers would rather be given standards than contraceptives. She describes a visit to a center for troubled teenagers during which a teacher asked what topic the girls wouldlike to discuss. They were disinterested in biology, infant care, and family planning, but their hands shot up when the teacher mentioned how to say no to a boyfriend without losing his love.[228]

Adolescents not only want help in overcoming pressure from their dates, but they also want to have their schools free from influences that will add to the pressure to be sexually active. In a recent Louis Harris poll, 87 percent of teens said they did not want comprehensive sexuality services in their schools. Sixty-seven percent said they did not even want such services in the vicinity of their schools.[229]

7. Will Abstinence Education Offend Parents Who Are Unmarried?

Some school officials are concerned that abstinence education will offend parents who are unmarried or who are living with someone to whom they are not married. Syndicated columnist William Raspberry responds:

> The half argument [against the teaching of morality in the schools] is that a classroom may include children whose own parents were never married and that it is, therefore, not possible to describe premarital or extramarital sex as immoral without condemning the parents of these children. But we are talking moral advice, not condemnation, and my guess is that even unwed parents would prefer their children postpone sexual activity at least until they are mature enough to handle it. In short, I don't see moral instruction as offensive to anyone.[230]

In addition, schools are in the business of teaching students the **best** way to do things, not necessarily the most comfortable. For example, in driver's education, schools teach students not to speed without worrying if their parents speed.

8. Are Parents Simply Concerned About Preventing Teenage Pregnancy Rather Than Preventing Promiscuity?

Some opponents of abstinence education claim that parents are more concerned about preventing pregnancy than they are about preventing promiscuity. When Louis Harris and Associates released the results of the poll commissioned by Planned Parenthood, Faye Wattleton, president of Planned Parenthood, announced that the poll showed most parents want schools to teach sex education. However, the poll also showed that 70 percent of adults want sex education to teach morals, and about the same percentage believe programs should urge students not to have sexual intercourse.[231]

Another major study has shown that parents want to pass along to their children three major values: self-restraint (i.e., premarital abstinence), compassion (i.e., empathy, caring), and commitment (i.e., marriage, fidelity).[232]

In light of the many misconceptions about abstinence education, it is important to examine what abstinence education is, how it is taught, and how effective it is.

C. THE DESIGN OF ABSTINENCE EDUCATION

When constructing an effective school program, it is important that the curriculum be morally based and philosophically sound. Various leaders of the abstinence movement have provided guidelines for the formation of appropriate materials.

Former Secretary of Education William Bennett advised:

- The approach cannot be values-neutral. It must teach children sexual restraint as a standard to uphold.

- It must teach that sex is not simply a physical or mechanical act. It involves emotions and feelings; some of them are ennobling, some are cheapening.

- Speak of sex in the context of the institution of marriage, fidelity, and commitment. Girls must be taught what it is to be a mother, as well as modesty and chastity. Boys must likewise be taught what it is to be a father, along with responsibility and readiness.

- Courses should welcome parents and other adults as allies.

- The school must pay attention to who is teaching the course. The teacher should serve as a good role model.[233]

Wanda Franz, associate professor of child development and family studies at West Virginia University, provides these guidelines for curriculum development:

- Develop materials that meet the needs of the targeted audience. Realize that too much information may do more harm than good.

- Develop a standard of maturity so that adolescents understand what the goal of their growth and development should be. Teens need to begin to value the recommendation to wait. While adolescents cannot fully understand these concepts, they can be helped to value them.

- Finally, develop sex education that will teach the best approach, not simply present an array of choices.[234]

The Family Research Council of America sets forth primary content guidelines that should also be considered:

- **Role of parents:** Parents are the first and most important educators. Programs should encourage parental participation, input, and review. They should have a clear method to stimulate parent-child discussion.

- **Abstinence:** Programs must clearly and unequivocally encourage premarital abstinence. Tell why abstinence is the wisest decision.

- **Contraception:** Advocating contraceptives among unmarried teens in an open classroom setting weakens the effectiveness of abstinence education. Mixed messages only confuse students.

- **Abortion:** Programs should focus on the physical, emotional, and spiritual problems abortion poses, and they should emphasize that abstinence prevents abortion.

- **Linking sex to marriage:** Programs should not suggest simply postponing intercourse. Instead, programs should link intercourse to marriage and teach that intercourse is a beautiful and meaningful experience when shared in the marital context.

- **Homosexuality:** Programs should not present homosexuality as an acceptable alternative lifestyle. Just like inappropriate heterosexual behavior, homosexuality has harmful physical, emotional, spiritual, and psychological consequences. (Note: Homosexual intercourse is also illegal in many states.)

- **Teacher:** The teacher must be of high moral character.[235]

Terrance Olson and Christopher Wallace, developers of the AANCHOR curriculum, offer these criteria for assessing family-life education curricula:

- Is the philosophy of the curriculum compatible with the basic educational philosophy of the school district? Does it promote the best interests of the individual, the student's family (past, present, and future), and society?

- Is it founded on principles basic to preventing and solving a wide range of problems (premarital teenage pregnancy, suicide, substance abuse, delinquency, etc.)?

- Does it avoid value stances that are either relativistic (where values are seen as preferences and are all of equal worth) or prescriptive (where a narrow, rule-oriented set of values is imposed)?

- Does it place responsibility on the individual to make responsible choices and not merely teach students to be willing to take responsibility for the consequences of any action?

- Does it support quality family living? That is, does it involve the family as a resource for making wise life decisions, and does it examine the relationship of individual identity to family relationships?

- What criteria for ethical assessment are provided? Does the curriculum encourage adolescents to learn to think and not simply memorize facts? Does it teach youths how to assess the value of a value?[236]

Besides criteria for assessing the content of curricula, Olson and Wallace list criteria for assessing the delivery of the content:

- Does it make the family context central to the delivery of ideas?

- Does it help students see the meaning of ethical principles?

- Does it demonstrate actions which promote the well-being of the individual, the family, and society?

- Does it avoid invading the private domain of the students' family experience?

- Does it acknowledge that the most fundamental analysis of behavior, across all disciplines that study human beings, is the moral-ethical dimension?[237]

D. THE NEED TO AVOID MIXED MESSAGES

In the vast array of sex education programs, there are materials that on the surface appear to meet the criteria for a morally based abstinence perspective. However, selection committees need to scrutinize all materials carefully so they will not inadvertently adopt items containing mixed messages.

For example, Planned Parenthood might appear to be an organization that favors adolescent abstinence because it has a pamphlet titled "Teensex" that tells young people it is "OK to say no way." But abstinence is being presented as one of several options; it is not being advocated as the **best** option. Planned Parenthood's Faye Wattleton said that her organization believes that "the answer to teen pregnancies lies not in preaching the return to a morality of an earlier time but in making teens have access to sex education and contraceptives." Waddleton went on to say:

> We are not going to be an organization promoting celibacy or chastity. Our concern is not to convey "shoulds" and "should nots," but to help young people make responsible decisions about their sexual relationships.... We've got to be more concerned about preventing teen pregnancies than we are about stopping sexual relationships.[238]

Another example of a program containing mixed messages is the curriculum *Human Sexuality: Values and Choices*. While it gives great emphasis to abstinence, it also contains a unit on contraception, and that portion is not designed to steer young people away from usage. The inclusion of the unit on contraception thus serves only to confuse adolescents.[239]

Postponing Sexual Involvement also contains confusing messages. While it is excellent for teaching young people the techniques of saying no, it does not give an absolute standard regarding premarital abstinence. Instead, teens are told to wait until they are mature or ready, which is a concept adolescents cannot comprehend; some might assume they are ready by age fifteen.[240]

The *School/Community Program for Sexual Risk Reduction Among Teens* operated in a high-risk area of a South Carolina county from October 1982 through September 1987. The educational objective of the program was to promote the postponement of sexual intercourse as the positive, preferred decision. Though contraception was presented as an option to teens who indicated they had chosen to become sexually active, it did not appear to be a major facet of the program.

Results show that the program did help to achieve a marked reduction in the teenage pregnancy rate; it went from 60 per 1,000 females before the program's inception to 25 per 1,000 females in 1985. The rate for comparison counties without the program showed an increase in teen pregnancies during the same time span.[241]

While educators might believe it is necessary to include a section on contraceptives for teens who are sexually active, they must realize that such an inclusion weakens the emphasis on abstinence. As has been shown in sections I, II, and III of this report, the contraceptive approach does not work: it has not reduced teen pregnancy or abortion; it has promoted promiscuity; it is not appropriate to adolescent cognitive development; and it confuses adolescent moral reasoning. On those bases alone, contraceptives should not be included in programs for teens.

Dr. Terrance Olson, who has tested the effectiveness of abstinence education, reports:

Since high school students are legal minors, it is appropriate that a family-centered approach be taken, and that abstinence be the prime approach, not even to be undermined by the idea that all other prevention options are equally defensible. . . . [O]ur efforts are less effective when teenagers are taught elsewhere that sexual decision-making is a grab-bag of equally defensible options.[242]

Other studies confirm the danger of mixed messages. The Louis Harris poll commissioned by Planned Parenthood showed that teens whose parents have discussed contraceptives have a greater likelihood to be sexually active than those whose parents do not discuss contraceptives in their sex education. The poll also showed that what applies at home applies in the classroom, as well. Teens who have a sex education course that discusses contraceptives have a 50 percent higher sexual activity rate than those who have had a sex education course omitting contraceptives or who have not had any sex education whatsoever. While Louis Harris and Associates say that their data do not show such a correlation, other statisticians, such as Professor Jacqueline Kasun of Humboldt State University, believe that the poll does show a relation between contraceptive education and sexual activity.[243]

Thus, the evidence indicates that mixed messages create problems in sex education, and effective curricula should advocate abstinence with no endorsements of contraceptives.

E. ESSENTIAL ELEMENTS IN ABSTINENCE EDUCATION

When developing or adopting an abstinence education program for the classroom, school officials must be careful in the definition used for abstinence. Unfortunately, some advocates of comprehensive sex education have redefined abstinence to only mean non-penetration, thus including oral sex, anal sex, mutual masturbation and external genital contact. Using this definition of abstinence, such people contend that it is **not** 100% effective because sperm released outside the vagina may enter the vagina, possibly resulting in impregnation. Also, including these activities in their definition, they claim the partners are not completely safe from contracting a sexually transmitted disease. Using this perspective, they claim that students who "abstain" are at risk and need to be taught about "safe sex." Such convoluted reasoning is being used to negate the real intent and effectiveness of abstinence education.[244] To prevent this misapplication, it is vital that abstinence be defined as the avoidance of sexual activity including intercourse, oral sex, anal sex, mutual masturbation and any genital contact which is sexually arousing.

In addition to considering the perspective regarding abstinence, people reviewing programs need to look for basic elements that contribute to a successful abstinence curriculum. Among these are:

(1) adolescent development: social, moral, cognitive, and physiological;

(2) individuality: interests, talents, and so on;

(3) family—past and present: importance in the development of character;

(4) responsibilities: to self, family, friends, co-workers, society;

(5) friendships: types, development of friendships, obligations;

(6) dating: setting standards for the type of person to date;

(7) infatuation versus love;

(8) consequences of premarital sex: physical (pregnancy, STDs, abortion) and psychological effects;

(9) freedoms that accompany premarital abstinence;

(10) techniques of saying no to sexual pressure;

(11) recognizing and resisting negative cultural influences;

(12) building relationships;

(13) making future plans;

(14) marriage;

(15) human reproduction;

(16) fetal development and childbirth;

(17) parenting;

(18) future family life.

As mentioned before, while many sex education programs cover these topics, it is important to present them in a value-based context and not from the perspective of a multitude of equally valid choices.

Also, it is important to assure that when certain subjects are covered (i.e., physiological development), girls and boys are separated out of sensitivity to students' shyness toward the subject. Further, if forced to sit through graphic viewings and discussions, adolescents may become desensitized to the subject. Unknowingly, educators would be removing modesty that is beneficial. Equally important, a mixed setting might inhibit the asking of important questions.

Finally, all material should be age-appropriate. Educational Guidance Institute has prepared an excellent detailed list of curriculum guidelines for each grade level. For further information, contact: Educational Guidance Institute, Inc., 927 S. Walter Reed Dr., Suite 4, Arlington, VA 22204, (703) 486-8313.

F. ABSTINENCE CURRICULA FOR THE PUBLIC SCHOOLS

There are several excellent, morally based abstinence curricula available for use in public schools. Corresponding with the guidelines and topics listed earlier, the curricula can be used easily by teachers, nurses, or whoever teaches the class. Each contains clearly stated objectives, carefully designed units, appropriate classroom exercises, and specific means of parental involvement. Curriculum descriptions are listed below, and the effectiveness of some of these programs is cited in the following section.

1. *AANCHOR* is an acronym for *An Alternative National Curriculum for Responsibility,* and it was designed for junior or senior high students in public schools under a grant from the OAPP. The curriculum is concerned with primary prevention in teaching youths to abstain from premarital intercourse. It is designed to help them learn to live responsible and wise lives by learning criteria by which to assess the quality of one's behavior, thoughts, and feelings.

AANCHOR consists of six modules: responsibility, ethical thinking, the family, communication, the law, and human reproduction.

Unlike most sex education courses, AANCHOR begins with a discussion of meaning, not merely the learning of facts. It uses case studies and role playing to help students develop moral decision-making abilities. It is not a values clarification approach; rather, it helps students realize why some choices are better than others. Parents are involved through parent-child discussions and homework assignments. For more information, contact Dr. Terrance Olson, Department of Family Sciences, Brigham Young University, Provo, Utah 84602, (801) 378-2069.

2. *Family Values and Sex Education: A Curriculum on Family and Citizenship for Middle School Students.* Designed for public junior high school health, family, or social studies classes, FVSE invites students to live in ways that promote their futures, strengthen their family relationships, and foster personal health and well-being. The curriculum lays a foundation of understanding quality family relationships; explores communication and decision-making; acknowledges the relationship of the family, society, and law; and discusses human reproduction, AIDS, and how to foster future families of high quality.

The curriculum has three modules: Family and Individual; Family Communication Skills and Family and The Next Generation (human reproduction). Parental involvement is central. Parent-teen worksheets are included to help guide family discussion of important topics and values.

The curriculum is not problem-centered. Instead, it focuses on how to live a wise and happy life, which helps young people to avoid crises. It offers positive ways to say no. The curriculum gives a clear endorsement of premarital abstinence. Contraceptive usage by unmarried teens is not promoted.

The curriculum was written by Terrance Olson, Ph.D., and Christopher Wallace, and was under the supervision of more than 100 academic and health experts. It can be obtained from Focus on the Family Publishing, Pomona, CA 91799, (714) 620-8500.

3. *Me, My World, My Future* is one of the newest programs receiving a grant from the OAPP. The curriculum contains fifteen lessons appropriate for public middle schools. This value-based program encourages the postponement of immediate gratification in exchange for healthier future goals in the areas of sexual activity, drugs, alcohol, and tobacco. Concrete learning activities are used to introduce the complex concepts of decision-making and communication.

To facilitate parental involvement, parent-teen communication worksheets accompany each lesson. The daily take-home sheets are designed to deepen the transmission of values from parents to teens by giving both the opportunity to discuss important subjects together. For more information, contact Teen-Aid, Inc., N. 1330 Calispel, Spokane, Washington 99201, (509) 466-8679 or (509) 328-2080.

4. *Sex Respect: The Option of True Sexual Freedom* is a curriculum developed through a grant under the Adolescent Family Life Act (AFLA), which is administered by the Office of Adolescent Pregnancy Programs (OAPP) of the U. S. Department of Health and Human Services.

The curriculum teaches that the best way to enjoy true sexual freedom in the long run is to say no to premarital sex. The units define human sexuality; recognize influences on sexual decision-making; identify emotional, psychological, and physical consequences of teenage sexual activity; discuss dating guidelines; teach how to say no; show how to change former sexual behavior; and explore the responsibilities of parenthood. Approximately ten hours of classroom time are needed to cover the material.

The curriculum includes three separate workbooks—one for students, one for teachers, and one for parents—that cover the same content and are used simultaneously. Originally intended for eighth and ninth graders, *Sex Respect* is now being used successfully in grades seven through eleven.

Sex Respect was written by Coleen Mast of Respect, Inc. The Committee on the Status of Women, directed by Kathleen Sullivan, is the grant recipient and field tester of the curriculum; the grant project is called Project Respect. Both Respect Incorporated and Project Respect have each developed separate high school curricula. Project Respect's new high school curriculum is *Facing Reality*.

For more information about the curricula, contact Respect, Inc., P.O. Box 349, Bradley, Illinois 60915-0349, (815) 932-8389, or Project Respect, Committee on the Status of Women, P.O. Box 97, Golf, Illinois 60029-0097, (312) 729-3298.

5. *Sexuality, Commitment, and Family* is a public high school curriculum that emphasizes the deep meaning of sexuality in the context of the family, of self-respect, of respect for others, and of respect and love for one's future spouse and children.

The curriculum is designed for a three-week program, which includes one day of introduction, one day of testing, and thirteen days of instruction. Areas of emphasis include: basic anatomy and maturational changes of adolescence; types of love; advantages of premarital abstinence; peer pressure; consequences of premarital sex; communication skills; and the fundamental purpose of marriage. Contraceptive risks are discussed, and students are steered away from usage.

Each lesson includes a worksheet to be taken home to keep parents informed about classroom lessons and to foster parent-teen communication. For more information, contact Teen-Aid, Inc., N. 1330 Calispel, Spokane, Washington 99201, (509) 466-8679 or (509) 328-2080.

G. EVALUATION OF ABSTINENCE EDUCATION

The abstinence education movement is beginning to have a positive effect on the views of adolescents toward premarital abstinence, in equipping young people to say no, and in helping to reduce the teenage pregnancy rate. While the results have not yet appeared in major journals, early reports are promising. Most studies are based on projects under the supervision and funding of the OAPP. Results from six of these projects are reported below.

1. *AANCHOR*. This project was tested from 1982 to 1987 in thirteen school districts in Utah, California, New Mexico, and Arizona.[245] Using a pre-test, post-test, and control group design (without random assignment), three statistically significant differences were obtained between post-test students receiving the AANCHOR curriculum and students receiving the standard school curriculum. After completing AANCHOR, students reported:
   (1) higher family strengths (loyalty, emotional support, cohesion),
   (2) more frequent discussions with parents about sexual values and beliefs, and
   (3) more abstinent attitudes regarding premarital sexual involvement.[246]

2. *Me, My World, My Future.* This curriculum has been used by over 2,500 schools. It was first tested at four junior high schools during the months of April and May of 1988. A pre-test and post-test questionnaire was administered, yielding 233 completed sets of data. The findings of this initial test indicated that the curriculum had statistically significant effects on a number of areas associated with teen sexual activity. Students indicated that they became more aware of the benefits of abstaining from sexual intercourse at their age, that they would be less likely to engage in intercourse before marriage, and that having sex as teenagers was against their values. They also were more likely to feel that teens who had had sexual intercourse would be better off to stop having sex and wait until they are married, and that waiting until marriage is the best way to avoid the problems which arise from promiscuous behavior. Students also indicated increased awareness of the negative consequences of teenage sexual behavior. The curriculum also had statistically significant effects on the students' view of when life begins in pregnancy as well as making them less likely to agree that sex was "OK" for teenagers if they were in love or if they used birth control.[247]

3. *Sex Respect.* Sex Respect has been adopted in over 1,000 school districts across the country. For example, from 1987 to 1989 it was taught to seventh graders at Lamar Junior High School in Lamar, Missouri. Of the approximately 450 students taking the program, there have been no pregnancies. School nurse Nancy Hughes attributes the success of the program to the values it teaches both girls and boys. As a result of the impact it is having on teenagers in the community, the school plans to continue teaching abstinence.[248]

   Though Lamar Junior High did not serve as an official part of the pilot program of Project Respect, the program has been tested extensively elsewhere. During its second year, the pilot program was used at 14 schools in 6 Midwestern states, with 1,841 students participating. The significant findings for the second year show:

   • Before taking the course, 36 percent of the students said sexual intercourse among teens is acceptable, provided no pregnancy results. Only 18 percent agreed after the course, and 65.5 percent disagreed.

   • Before the course, 20 percent said sexual urges are "always" controllable, and 62 percent said they are "sometimes." Afterward, 39 percent said "always," and 51 percent said "sometimes."

   • Before the course, 35 percent said there are "a lot" of benefits to waiting until marriage for sexual intercourse. After taking the course, 58 percent agreed.[249]

Bar graphs help to illustrate many of the items tested in Project Respect. Refer to Tables 24-28.[250]

Effectiveness of the Project Respect Program

Table 24
Dating in mixed groups is less likely to lead to sexual activity.

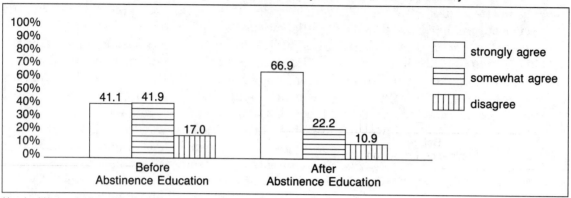

Table 25
Do TV and movies influence what you do on a date?

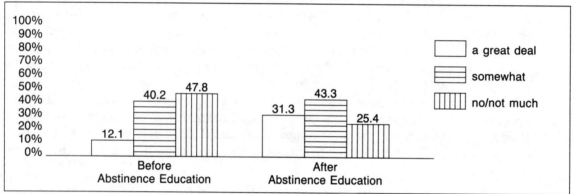

Table 26
Is the sex act all right for unmarried teens as long as no pregnancy results?

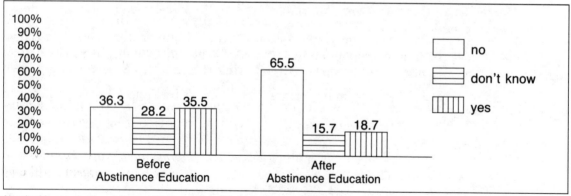

Table 27
Do you think there are benefits to waiting until marriage for sexual intercourse?

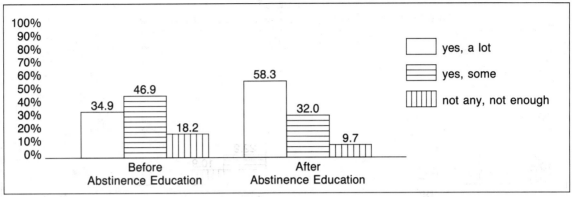

Table 28
Once a teen has had sex outside of marriage, he/she would benefit
by deciding to stop having sex and wait till marriage

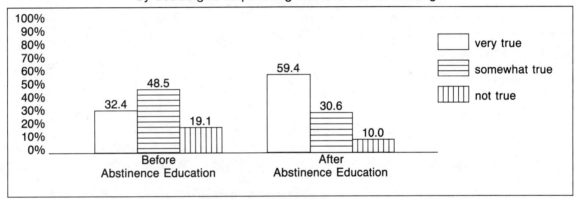

4. *Sexuality, Commitment, and Family.* This curriculum has been purchased by 2,500 school districts across the country. While it has not been officially tested, one case study reveals the extent to which it affected a community.

The city of San Marcos, California, made headlines across the country when it was revealed that during the 1983-84 school year, 178 junior high and high school girls (1 in 5 girls) had become pregnant. Only 9 pregnancies ended in childbirth; the others miscarried or were aborted.

School officials and parents decided not to ignore the crisis, nor to join the increasing number of schools promoting contraceptives. In a strong consensus, community leaders opted for a more structured approach that would seek to change attitudes and behavior. The school district developed lessons on study skills and adopted the abstinence curriculum *Sexuality, Commitment, and Family.*[251]

San Marcos Junior High reported the extent to which its program affected students in the first two years, as shown in Table 29.[252]

Table 29

Impact of Abstinence Program on Teen Pregnancies and Grades

Category	1984–85	1986–87
Students with 4.0 GPA	2.2%	4.5%
Students with 3.0 GPA	34.6%	35.3%
Attendance rate	98.6%	98.9%
Percent of students in lowest quartile of CTBS	16.4%	11.7%
Number of girls reported pregnant at our high school	147	20

Source: Teen Aid, Inc., N. 1330 Calispel, Spokane, WA 99201.

In a letter to Teen-Aid, which developed the abstinence curriculum used at the school, the principal of San Marcos Junior High said, "Our staff, students, and parents are excited about the program. You have just cause to be very proud of your Teen-Aid program. It fits perfectly with what we are attempting to do. Based upon the interest in our program from other communities, it is obvious many communities are looking for what Teen-Aid is offering."[253]

5. *Teen Choice.* Since December 1987, Teen Choice has given presentations to over 1700 students in Fairfax and Arlington counties in Virginia. Currently, Teen Choice is giving a fifty-minute program entitled "Reasonable Reasons to Wait," which includes a presentation of the developmental branches of adolescence (social, intellectual, moral, physical, emotional), the bridges to adulthood, the advantages of premarital abstinence, the role of sexual intercourse in marriage, and secondary virginity.

The presentation has been shown to significantly affect students' opinions. Approximately 700 students were given a pre-test and post-test, thus measuring the short-term impact of the presentation. The results are summarized below. Evaluation plans call for a future administration of a delayed post-test, perhaps six months after the presentation, to assess longer-term impact on student attitudes. For information about the program, contact Teen Choice, Educational Resource Center, P.O. Box 284, Falls Church, Virginia 22046, (703) 532-9455.

The results as of July 1988 are shown in Table 30.[254] Considering that the changes occurred after a relatively short presentation, the figures suggest that teenagers respond favorably to an abstinence message.

Table 30
Effectiveness of the Teen Choice Program

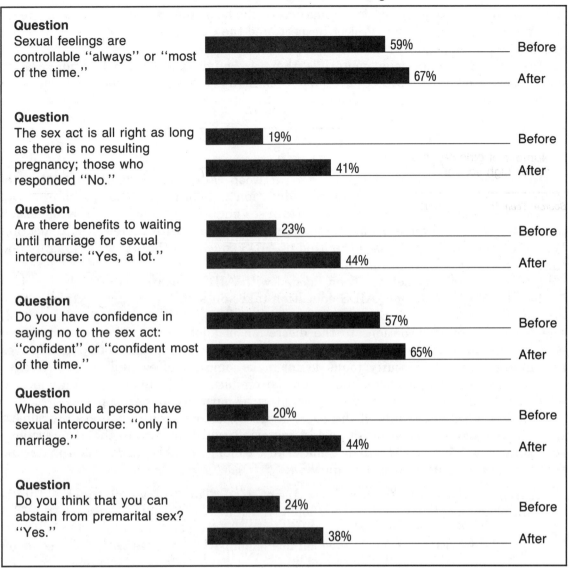

Question		
Sexual feelings are controllable "always" or "most of the time."	59%	Before
	67%	After
The sex act is all right as long as there is no resulting pregnancy; those who responded "No."	19%	Before
	41%	After
Are there benefits to waiting until marriage for sexual intercourse: "Yes, a lot."	23%	Before
	44%	After
Do you have confidence in saying no to the sex act: "confident" or "confident most of the time."	57%	Before
	65%	After
When should a person have sexual intercourse: "only in marriage."	20%	Before
	44%	After
Do you think that you can abstain from premarital sex? "Yes."	24%	Before
	38%	After

Adapted from data by Teen Choice.

H. ABSTINENCE EDUCATION MEDIA

Educators need to seek out appropriate audiovisual materials that can be used in conjunction with other classroom resources. As with other materials, audiovisual aids should promote abstinence and should be appealing to adolescents.

As part of the national *Why Wait? Media Campaign,* Josh McDowell Ministries has developed a variety of audiovisual resources designed for teens and parents. Topics addressed in the films include dating standards, the importance of waiting, how to say no, building relationships, and other issues related to adolescent sexuality. Some films are designed for the public school classroom, and others are more appropriate in church settings. Many of these are available on free loan for public school showings. For more information, contact Gospel Films, Box 455, Muskegon, Michigan, 49443, (800) 253-0413. To obtain a complete list of the *Why Wait?* resources (cassette tapes, books, and other aids), contact Why Wait?, Josh McDowell Ministries, Box 1000, Dallas, Texas

75221, (214) 907-1000. To make a direct purchase, contact their Illinois distribution center at (800) 222-JOSH.

Other organizations have also produced excellent abstinence media, including Teen-Aid, Womanity, Respect, Inc., Project Respect, and the Couple to Couple League. See the list of films in Appendix H of this report.

In addition to audiovisual materials, there are numerous pamphlets, audiocassette tapes, books, and other resources available from many organizations that are involved in abstinence education. See the appendixes in the back of this report for details.

I. AIDS EDUCATION

In October 1986, then Surgeon General Koop called for the implementation of kindergarten through twelfth grade sex education to help reduce the spread of AIDS. Having been shown the explicitness of certain sex education materials, Dr. Koop issued a new statement a few months later. In a joint press release with Secretary of Education William Bennett, Koop stressed the kind of AIDS education that must be taught—one that encourages premarital abstinence and marital fidelity.[255]

Since then, the market has been flooded with AIDS educational material. Just as in the case of sex education, AIDS education takes on a variety of perspectives. There are those programs that discuss safe sex, refer briefly to abstinence, are values-neutral, and leave the lifestyle options to the discretion of adolescents. As has been shown earlier in this report, condom usage is not safe sex, the advocacy of contraceptives actually promotes promiscuity, teens do not make logical choices, and mixed messages are detrimental. Furthermore, progressive sex education during the latency period (elementary school years) can cause psychological harm to young people.

Because of the timeliness of the AIDS issue, educators need to address the subject in the classroom, but they need to select materials which adhere to the same criteria set forth for value-based abstinence materials. Among the AIDS education materials that meet these criteria are the following:

1. *Who Do You Listen To? Sex in the Age of AIDS*. This thirty-minute AIDS film is intended for public secondary schools. Written with a positive message, the film presents a drama in a classroom setting. The teacher's lecture and student-teacher interaction contain medical facts about AIDS. Scenes with adolescents on dates who are struggling with and making moral decisions help to underscore the right choices teens should make. A visit to an AIDS hospice helps viewers realize the tragedy of the disease and the importance of changing promiscuous behavior. Premarital abstinence and marital fidelity are emphasized.

   The film is available on free loan to public schools through Gospel Films, Box 455, Muskegon, Michigan 49443, (800) 253-0413. Film details can be obtained from Why Wait?, Josh McDowell Ministries, Box 1000, Dallas, Texas 75221, (214) 907-1000.

2. *AIDS—Learn and Live*. This twenty-five-minute video is intended for seventh through tenth grade public school students. Done in the form of a news documentary, it contains interviews with physicians, teens, and AIDS victims. The video also contains some scenarios in which teens act out refusal skills. The topics addressed in the video are premarital abstinence, condom failure, epidemiology of the HIV virus (how it works and how it spreads), and how to say no. Accompanying the tape is an update on the medical facts regarding AIDS. A useful accompanying pamphlet entitled "Is There Real Safe Sex?" is available from the producers.

   For information, contact Teen-Aid, Inc., N. 1330 Calispel, Spokane, Washington 99201, (509) 466-8679 or (509) 328-2080.

3. *AIDS: Suddenly Sex Has Become Very Dangerous (revised edition).* This is a three-tape series that includes:

   (1) a tape for teens containing dramatic segments;
   (2) a teachers' and parents' version that has the same material as the teen tape, along with introductory and concluding messages for parental and teacher preview; and
   (3) a medical facts tape about the AIDS virus, with simple, straightforward information obtained through interviews with medical experts.

   The series promotes premarital abstinence, marital fidelity, avoidance of intimate kissing, and avoidance of drug abuse. For more information, contact Goodday Video, 115 N. Esplanade St., Cuero, Texas 77954, (800) 221-1426.

4. *AIDS: A Risky Business for Everyone.* This program was developed by Coleen Mast as a supplement to the *Sex Respect* curriculum. Like *Sex Respect,* it comes in three separate workbooks: one for teachers, one for students, and one for parents.

   The program discusses the high fatality rate of AIDS, the levels of AIDS infection, the transmission of the virus, and the prevention of AIDS through avoiding drugs, premarital sex, extramarital sex, and homosexual activity. It refutes the myth of safe sex via condoms.

   The curriculum includes current medical data, discussion questions, case studies, and practical advice designed for junior or senior high students. For more information, contact Respect, Inc., P.O. Box 349, Bradley, Illinois 60915-0349, (815) 932-8389.

5. *AIDS and Young People.* This is a booklet written by Robert Redfield, M.D., of the Walter Reed Army Institute of Research, and Wanda Franz, associate professor of family resources, West Virginia University. It covers the definition of AIDS, the origin of the virus, how people die from AIDS, the means of transmission, the extent of the disease, the categories of people infected, tests for AIDS, how to avoid getting AIDS, and the myth of safe sex.

   The booklet is designed as a module for classroom usage. For more information, contact the Coalition for Appropriate Sex Education, Concerned Women for America, 370 L'Enfant Promenade S.W., Suite 800, Washington, D.C. 20024, (800) 458-8797, or Project Respect, Committee on the Status of Women, Box 97, Golf, Illinois 60029-0097, (312) 729-3298.

6. *AIDS and the Education of Our Children: Guide for Parents and Teachers.* This booklet, developed by the U. S. Department of Education, provides a description of AIDS, symptoms, the incurability of the disease, the means of transmission, teenage risk behavior, the limits of information and education, and means to help protect young people. It clearly stresses premarital abstinence. For more information, contact the U. S. Department of Education, 400 Maryland Ave. S.W., Room 4019, Washington, D.C. 20202, (202) 732-4024.

7. *Will "Safe Sex" Education Effectively Combat AIDS?* This informal paper was developed by the Department of Education as an abstract of research showing the fallacy of safe sex. It cites seventy-eight sources that show why condoms are not effective in preventing the transmission of the AIDS virus, and why premarital abstinence and marital fidelity are important.

   This paper is an excellent resource for people who must decide which perspective will be presented in a classroom. For more information, contact the U. S. Department of Education, 400 Maryland Ave. S.W., Room 4019, Washington, D.C. 20202, (202) 732-4024.

8. *Living Safely in the Age of AIDS.* This publication is a curriculum developed for public school usage. The manual is designed for use by both instructor and student,providing detailed lesson plans for ten sessions. Among the topics included are the definition of AIDS, the seriousness of the disease, a description of the body's immune system, the virus and how it attacks the body, its transmission, attitudes and actions which foster AIDS, preventing risk and infection, love and marriage, and fighting AIDS effectively.

Each lesson includes description, review questions and discussion questions. For more information, contact: National AIDS Prevention Institute, P.O. Box 2500, Culpeper, VA 22701, (703) 825-4040.

J. TEACHER TRAINING

When enrolled in college, most teachers did not receive any training about the value of abstinence education or how to teach it. If they received any instruction in human sexuality, it was probably in the form of contraceptive sex education. So when teachers want to adopt an abstinence perspective, they often feel unprepared. Also, when schools adopt an abstinence perspective, some teachers are skeptical about the approach and need to discover that it is a teachable, effective method. For those reasons, schools should seek out teacher training that is geared toward abstinence education.

Most organizations that have developed abstinence materials can also send trainers for intensive workshops or in-service training. In addition, some groups offer videotapes of their training. For information about teacher training, contact the organizations that produce abstinence materials.

In many cases, teachers can receive state-approved credits for advanced academic training they obtain at such workshops. Personnel who are coordinating a workshop in a community should check with their respective state education agency and complete the necessary application months prior to a workshop.

Teachers generally respond favorably after going through abstinence training. At the end of a *Sex Respect* workshop, one teacher responded, "It gives me confidence in myself that I can go back to the students and give them this program with the understanding that it will work if they want it to." Another said that it "will make a great deal of difference in how kids make their decisions about premarital sex." The training helps educators see why abstinence education is superior to contraceptive education. As one educator remarked, it is "quite the opposite of the programs I have become familiar with over the last five years. It's different in the sense of encouraging teens to abstain from sex until marriage instead of saying, 'If you want to, here's what you can use to prevent pregnancy.' I love this program."[256]

An excellent resource for teachers is the book by teacher trainer Pat Socia, *Teaching True Abstinence Sex Education.* It is available from Project Respect, P.O. Box 97, Golf, Illinois 60029-0097, (312) 729-3298.

VI. *PARENTAL INVOLVEMENT*

Parental involvement in educating children about sexuality is essential in reducing teenage promiscuity, fostering a proper perspective on the role of sex in marriage, and promoting a wholesome family life for future generations. In *Teen Pregnancy: What Is Being Done? A State-by-State Look,* the minority members of the U. S. House Select Committee on Children, Youth, and Families affirmed the importance of parental involvement:

> The time has come to stop blaming the problems of teen pregnancy on the incorrigibility of our children or the ills of society. Our children have only us for guidance; and we are responsible for the condition of our society. The real path back to a sane and effective policy to prevent teen pregnancies is not an easy one, but it is the only one that will work. It is also the only one that most of us would choose for our own sons and daughters. The path does not circumvent the family, but leads straight to the heart of it. It encourages communication between parents and children and is built on the firm foundation of parents' values, beliefs, and ambitions for their children.[257]

One of the major aims of the Adolescent Family Life Demonstration Projects is to promote family involvement in sex education. Programs funded by the OAPP must comply with the clause that states the purpose:

> ...to find effective means, within the context of the family, of reaching adolescents before they become sexually active in order to maximize the guidance and support available to adolescents from parents and other family members, and to promote self-discipline and other prudent approaches to the problem of adolescent premarital sexual relations, including adolescent pregnancy.[258]

A. FORMS OF PARENTAL INVOLVEMENT

Parental involvement can take on various forms and degrees of participation. The more the involvement, the greater the effectiveness in positively influencing young people. Some of the ways parents can take part are as follows.

1. *Parents as the primary educators.* The best form of parental involvement is for parents to be the primary educators. Because parents often feel inadequate or uncomfortable about this responsibility, they may need training. It is better for schools to help train parents than to usurp the role of parents as teachers.

2. *Parents serving on school committees.* Parents can also take part in the selection and review of materials for schools. To accomplish this, parents should be elected or appointed to special committees within the school district, at particular schools, and in parent-teacher associations. Those serving on committees should play a major role in setting criteria, forming objectives, selecting materials, and voting on all relevant issues pertaining to sex education, counseling about sexuality, and health services for teens.

3. *Parental questionnaires and public hearings.* All parents should be given questionnaires that allow them to provide input to the school's sex education committee, and the data collected should have a major effect on committee decisions. Also, public hearings can increase parental awareness and input.

4. *Parental preview.* Another form of parental involvement should be the previewing of all policies, programs, and materials by all parents. This should be done months prior to an intended date for classroom implementation of materials. By doing this in advance, schools will have sufficient time to remove materials that are deemed objectionable and to find better resources.

Some developers of abstinence materials have prepared videotapes for parental previewing sessions. Contact the respective publishers to find out if such tapes are available.

5. *Parental attendance in the classroom.* Parents can also attend during the actual classroom presentation of sex education. *Fertility Appreciation for Families* and *Learning About Myself and Others* are two examples of programs that **require** parental participation. Usually, these programs are offered in the evenings or on weekends so that parental attendance will be convenient. Some programs or schools make parental attendance optional. If a program or school **forbids** parental attendance, parents have good reason to question the appropriateness of the program.

6. *Parent-teen discussion sheets or workbooks for home.* Involvement can also come through take-home worksheets distributed to teens at the end of each lesson. The highlight the topics addressed in the classroom and list questions that can help guide parent-teen discussion. Some curricula offer an entire workbook for parents.

The importance of this method is that it helps to reinforce the family's immediate and long-term influences on their child's moral reasoning and value system as it is being developed. Also, by receiving a handout for each session, or workbook for the entire course, parents will not have to depend solely on their child's recall of what occurred in the classroom. Finally, the handouts or workbook can list sensitive topics that were not addressed in the classroom but need to be discussed between parents and teens.

Among the curricula that use parent-teen communication worksheets are *Family Values and Sex Education; Sexuality, Commitment, and Family; Me, My World, My Future*; and *AANCHOR*. The curriculum *Sex Respect* uses an entire workbook for parents rather than a series of take-home sheets.

7. *Parental permission forms.* The last and weakest type of parental involvement is a parental permission form for student participation in sex education. For all federally funded programs, this is required by law according to the Education Amendment of 1978.[259] Compliance is usually handled by sending home a permission slip that allows parents to excuse their children from sex education classes. This approach is sometimes labeled as "negative parental consent." Many states and local school districts have developed similar policies.

While it is important for parents to have the right to remove their children from such classes, there are many drawbacks to this procedure. One is that parents often do not receive the slips, and unless the slips are returned to the schools, students end up attending programs that parents might find objectionable. Another is that the system can create friction between parent and child. Teens whose parents remove them often become the real or perceived objects of ridicule from peers and teachers, and then they blame their parents for letting them become targets of criticism. A third drawback is that the procedure can brand some parents as troublemakers, thereby making it difficult for them to have a positive influence on the educational system.

While parental permission is important, there is a better way of handling it. Rather than using a form that only allows opting out, the form should be written so that unless the form is returned with a signature of approval, a student will not be allowed to attend the class. This method is "opting in," sometimes called "positive parental consent." While it, too, might cause some students to become objects of ridicule, it reduces that likelihood.

Another way of handling parental permission, particularly in a school district in which some people insist that the school offer contraceptive information, is to teach an abstinence-only perspective in the regular classroom program. Then offer a before-school or take-home lesson on contraceptives, only allowing students to participate whose parents have signed written forms indicating that they want their children to receive this instruction. This practice was implemented at San Marcos Junior High (San Marcos, California), and of the 450-500 students that have taken the abstinence program, less than 20 (4%) of the students' parents have indicated that they want their children to be taught about contraceptives.[260]

Unfortunately, most sex education programs across the country use only the permission form, which is a superficial means of parental involvement.

B. PARENT-TRAINING WORKSHOPS

As stated earlier, the best form of parental involvement is for parents to be the primary educators of their children. Many schools would like to see this, but they are unsure how to make it happen. One way is for schools or community groups to set up a workshop that teaches parents how to fulfill their role. There are excellent programs that schools can use to accomplish this goal. Among them are the following:

1. *Fertility Appreciation for Families.* From 1983-87, Family of the Americas developed and field tested a family-centered educational program that promotes chastity, respect for life, and authentic moral values. Under a grant from the OAPP, it was developed to strengthen the family as the first and best source of education in human sexuality. The program features an educational process based on traditional family values; development of communication among family members; helping parents to identify and transmit values to their children; reinforcing parental confidence in helping children through puberty and sexual decision making; providing thorough information about child and adolescent development; and presenting the latest information about the anatomy and physiology of human fertility. In this program, parents and teens attend together.

    For information about the program, contact Family for the Americas Foundation, 1150 Lovers Lane, Mandeville, Louisiana 71448, (504) 626-7724.

2. *A Parent's Guide: Teaching Responsible Sexual Behavior.* This parent workshop (also developed under a grant from the OAPP) is ten hours long and is divided into five two-hour sessions: an overview, sexuality information, making the best choice, supporting the best choice, and tools for parenting. A trainer's manual and parental handouts are available so that schools or groups can conduct the workshop in their communities. For more information, contact Teen-Aid, Inc., N. 1330 Calispel, Spokane, Washington 99201, (509) 466-8679 or (509) 328-2080.

3. *Challenge Program.* The Educational Guidance Institute's *Challenge Program* is conducted outside of school and taught to parents and teens in four two-hour sessions. Themes stressed in the program are the value of human sexuality within the context of marriage and a credible rationale for premarital abstinence.

    The program is being used in Washington, D.C., Maryland, and Virginia. Its uniqueness is that it draws upon existing materials from *Sex Respect* and Teen-Aid and adapts the materials to a particular community's needs. The program shows that an abstinence message can be presented in various ways and that the philosophical foundation of abstinence is the key to effectiveness in sex education.

    Under the direction of Margaret Whitehead and Onalee McGraw, Ph.D., the Institute has put together a team of professionals who are influencing their community. While the Institute does not offer a curriculum for usage across the country, it has shown how to adapt curricula for a particular community, especially where schools are unlikely to implement abstinence education. The Institute has also developed an excellent list of curriculum guidelines for each grade level. Their advice is helpful in determining what is age-appropriate for students.

For a brief description of their work, contact the Educational Guidance Institute, Inc., 927 S. Walter Reed Dr., Suite 4, Arlington, Virginia 22204, (703) 486-8313.

4. *How to Help Your Child Say No to Sexual Pressure.* This is an eight-part video series for parents of teens and preteens that addresses the youth culture, why youths say yes to sex, balancing rules and relationships, how to equip your child with reasons to wait, how to teach your child to say no, and how to build bridges of communication between parents and teens.

The video curriculum comes with a leader's manual, lesson discussion leaflets, and a companion book with the same title as the video series. While the series does contain religiously based insights, it is a positive message that can be used in a general setting without controversy. For more information, contact Why Wait?, Josh McDowell Ministries, Box 1000, Dallas, Texas 75221, (214) 907-1000.

C. EVALUATION OF PARENTAL INVOLVEMENT

Studies have shown that the more involved parents are with their teenagers, the more likely the teens will be protected from the problems of premarital pregnancy.[261]

Laws regarding parental involvement have also been shown to help reduce teenage pregnancies. For example, in 1981 Minnesota implemented a law requiring parental notification before abortions could be performed on minors, and from 1980 to 1983, there was a 32 percent reduction in teen pregnancies, a 23.4 percent reduction in teen births, and a 40 percent reduction in teen abortions.[262]

Even laws preventing physicians from dispensing contraceptives to minors without parental consent can improve the teenage pregnancy problem. For example, when England banned doctors from prescribing contraceptives to minors, the numbers of pregnancies, births, and abortions all decreased.[263]

Apart from laws, educational programs that involve parents as the primary educators of their children have been shown to help reduce the incidence of teen pregnancy. The effectiveness of such programs is described below.

1. *AANCHOR.* The *AANCHOR* curriculum has also been shown to have a positive influence in promoting family and adolescent communication regarding sexuality. After taking it, students reported higher family strengths (loyalty), greater discussion with parents about sexual values and beliefs, and more abstinent attitudes regarding premarital involvement.[264]

2. *Challenge Program.* Educational Guidance Institute's *Challenge Program* brought parents and teens together for a four-hour session. At the beginning of the program, 51% of the parents felt prepared to teach their children about sexuality; at the end, 91% did. At the beginning, 48% felt very confident as the moral teachers of their children; at the end, 71% did. Before the program, only 3% of the parents had discussed dating guidelines with their children; at the end, 40% had.

Communication between parents and teens increased significantly on many topics, such as talking about the difference between love and infatuation, discussing sexual pressures on teens, and discussing the relationship between freedom and responsibility.

Table 31
Attitudes of Young People About Sex and Sexuality*

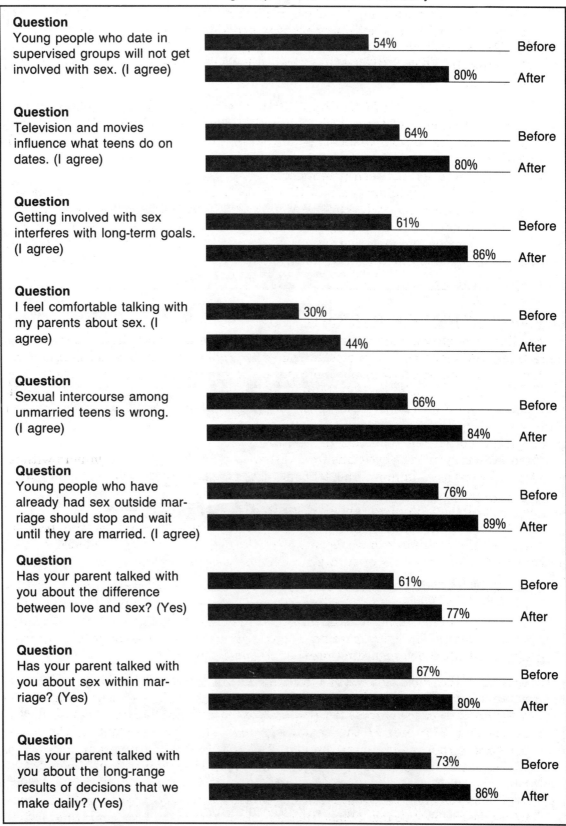

Question
Young people who date in supervised groups will not get involved with sex. (I agree)
- 54% Before
- 80% After

Question
Television and movies influence what teens do on dates. (I agree)
- 64% Before
- 80% After

Question
Getting involved with sex interferes with long-term goals. (I agree)
- 61% Before
- 86% After

Question
I feel comfortable talking with my parents about sex. (I agree)
- 30% Before
- 44% After

Question
Sexual intercourse among unmarried teens is wrong. (I agree)
- 66% Before
- 84% After

Question
Young people who have already had sex outside marriage should stop and wait until they are married. (I agree)
- 76% Before
- 89% After

Question
Has your parent talked with you about the difference between love and sex? (Yes)
- 61% Before
- 77% After

Question
Has your parent talked with you about sex within marriage? (Yes)
- 67% Before
- 80% After

Question
Has your parent talked with you about the long-range results of decisions that we make daily? (Yes)
- 73% Before
- 86% After

*These results are from the first phase of a multi-year project of the Educational Guidance Institute, Inc. The data are based on the responses of 53 young people, ages 11 to 18, who were tested at two points in time, the first prior to a two-week program on sexual values, and the second at the conclusion of the program. The above distributions of responses are statistically different between the first and second testings (based on paired t-tests).

The young people in the program showed evidence of increased communication with parents on sexual matters and greater understanding of the reasons to value premarital abstinence. Also, teens said that they were now more comfortable talking to their parents about sex, talking with parents about how to behave on a date, and that sex might interfere with long-term goals.

Tables 31 and 32 show the before-and-after results of the program sponsored by Educational Guidance Institute.[265]

Table 32
Attitudes of Parents about Sex and Sexuality*

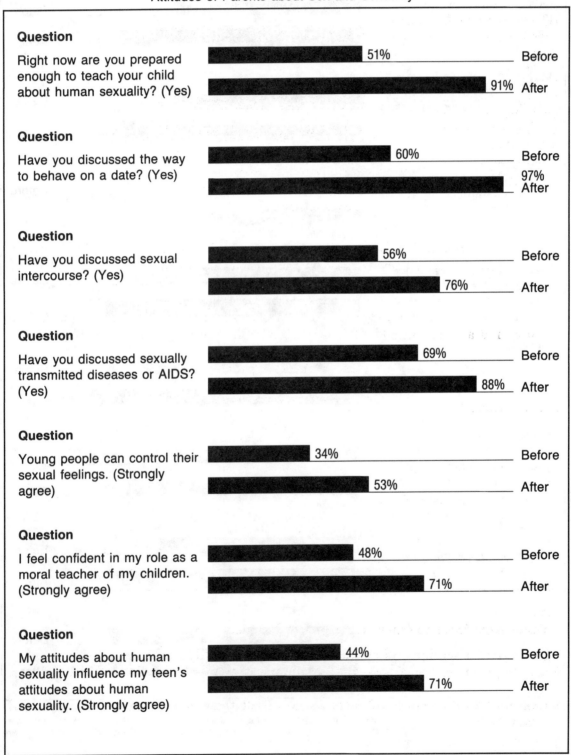

Question

Right now are you prepared enough to teach your child about human sexuality? (Yes)

51% — Before
91% — After

Question

Have you discussed the way to behave on a date? (Yes)

60% — Before
97% After

Question

Have you discussed sexual intercourse? (Yes)

56% — Before
76% — After

Question

Have you discussed sexually transmitted diseases or AIDS? (Yes)

69% — Before
88% — After

Question

Young people can control their sexual feelings. (Strongly agree)

34% — Before
53% — After

Question

I feel confident in my role as a moral teacher of my children. (Strongly agree)

48% — Before
71% — After

Question

My attitudes about human sexuality influence my teen's attitudes about human sexuality. (Strongly agree)

44% — Before
71% — After

Table 32 (continued)

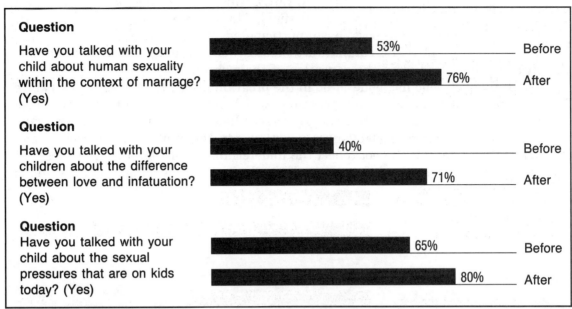

Question		
Have you talked with your child about human sexuality within the context of marriage? (Yes)	53%	Before
	76%	After

Question		
Have you talked with your children about the difference between love and infatuation? (Yes)	40%	Before
	71%	After

Question		
Have you talked with your child about the sexual pressures that are on kids today? (Yes)	65%	Before
	80%	After

These results are from the first phase of a multi-year project of the Educational Guidance Institute, Inc. The data are based on the responses of 54 parents of youth who were tested at two points in time, the first prior to a two-week program on sexual values, and the second at the conclusion of the program. The above distributions of responses are statistically different between the first and second testings (based on paired t-tests).

3. *Fertility Appreciation for Families.* First described in section VI.B. of this report, this program was demonstrated in four test centers from 1983 to 1987. It was presented to more than 6,000 participants, including 3,678 adolescents and 2,478 parents. Of this group, 630 adolescents were questioned one year after their participation in the program. Results show that only three pregnancies had occurred among the 630 adolescents. Table 33 shows that the pregnancy rate for the participants is roughly 5 percent of the national average.[266]

Table 33
Teenage Pregnancy 15–19-year-olds

Study	Number of Pregnancies
Alan Guttmacher Institute	96 per 1000
Planned Parenthood Clinic (Weed & Olsen, 1986)	113 per 1000
Fertility Appreciation for Families	4 per 1000

Other significant findings of the project include:

(1) increased knowledge and appreciation of human fertility among participants;
(2) increased confidence of parents in communicating this knowledge to their children; and
(3) increased willingness of adolescents to consult their parents with questions about sexuality.[267]

4. *Learning About Myself and Others (LAMO).* This program has been widely used with good results in and around Pittsfield, Massachusetts, since 1975. At least 6,000 girls and 4,000 boys have participated in the program during their elementary school years. Parental attendance was required, and parents became involved as co-leaders in the education of their children.

Of the girls who had gone through the program from 1975 to 1987, only twelve were reported to have become pregnant, which represents about one per school year. In the same community, among girls who had not gone through the program, the number of pregnant teens was about twenty to twenty-five per school year. While these statistics do not reflect the undetermined number of pregnancies that ended in abortion, the informal analysis shows that the program is having a positive influence.[268]

VII. *A FINAL NOTE*

Moving into the 1990s, parents, educators, clergy, health care workers, community leaders, and legislators need to cooperate in their efforts to help young people build a positive foundation for human sexuality, marriage, and family life. The highest moral standards should not be cast aside as in the past two decades. When allowed to be the center of a program, they serve as the framework of effective sex education.

Decision makers are beginning to scrutinize the proposals of special interest groups and are seeking more effective and less expensive solutions to the teenage sexuality crisis. Enough evidence is becoming available to help them make better choices.

ENDNOTES

I. FAMILY PLANNING PROGRAMS FOR ADOLESCENTS

1. Population Reference Bureau, *World Population Growth and Response: 1965-75—A Decade of Global Action* (Washington, D.C.: Population Reference Bureau, April 1976), p. 184, as cited in Jacqueline Kasun, "The State and Adolescent Sexual Behavior," in Joseph R. Peden and Fred R. Glahe, eds., *The American Family and the State* (San Francisco: Pacific Research Institute for Public Policy, 1986), p. 329.

2. Peden and Glahe, eds., *The American Family*, p. 330.

3. 42 U. S. Code, sec. 602(a), as cited in Peden and Glahe, eds., *The American Family*, p. 329.

4. Commission of Population Growth and the American Future, *Research Reports I* (Washington, D.C.: Government Printing Office, 1972), as cited in Peden and Glahe, eds., *The American Family*, p. 330.

5. Planned Parenthood Federation of America Five Year Plan, 1976-80, pp. ii-10.

6. *11 Million Teenagers: What Can Be Done About the Epidemic of Adolescent Pregnancies in the United States* (New York: Guttmacher Institute, 1976).

7. Gilbert Steiner, *The Futility of Family Policy* (Washington, D.C.: Brookings Institution, 1981), pp. 80-85, as cited in Peden and Glahe, eds., *The American Family*, p. 333.

8. *Planned Births, the Future of the Family and the Quality of American Life* (Planned Parenthood, et al, June 1977), pp. 3, 18-19, 30, as cited in Peden and Glahe, eds., *The American Family*, p. 333.

9. Peden and Glahe, eds., *The American Family*, pp. 333-334.

10. *Teenage Pregnancy: The Problem That Hasn't Gone Away* (New York: Guttmacher Institute, 1981).

11. Office of Population Affairs, *The Adolescent Family Life Demonstration Projects: Program and Evaluation Summaries* (Washington, D.C.: Office of Population Affairs, HHS, 1987), pp. i-ii, 288-303.

12. Elise F. Jones, et al, "Teenage Pregnancy in Developed Countries: Determinants and Policy Implications," *Family Planning Perspectives* 17 (March/April 1985), pp. 53-62.

13. See, for example, *Time*, 11/24/86; *Newsweek*, 2/16/87; and *Reader's Digest*, March 1987.

14. American College of Obstetricians and Gynecologists, pamphlet entitled "The Facts: What You Need to Know About Contraceptives to Make the Right Choice."

15. Committee on Adolescence, "Contraception and the Media," *Pediatrics* (September 1986), pp. 535-536, and "AAP Guidelines: School-Based Health Clinics," *AAP News*, April 1987, p. 7.

16. C. D. Hayes, *Risking the Future: Adolescent Sexuality, Pregnancy, and Childbearing* (National Research Council, 1987), pp. 7-10, 165.

17. *Informing Social Change* (New York: Guttmacher Institute, 1980), p. 7, as cited in Peden and Glahe, eds., *The American Family*, p. 354.

18. Jacqueline Kasun, "Teenage Pregnancy: Media Effects Versus Facts," (Stafford, Va.: American Life League, 1986), p. 3.

19. Jacqueline Kasun, "Teenage Pregnancy: What Comparisons Among States and Countries Show," (Stafford, Virg.: American Life League, 1986).

20. Faye Wattleton, *The Humanist* (July/August 1986), p. 7.

21. U. S. Department of Health and Human Services, fact sheet "Adolescent Pregnancy and Childbearing."

22. Kasun, "Teenage Pregnancy: What Comparisons Among States and Countries Show," p. 6.

23. Testimony before the U. S. Senate Committee on Labor and Human Resources, March 31, 1981, as cited in Peden and Glahe, eds., *The American Family*, p. 355.

24. Joseph A. Olsen and Stan Weed, "Effects of Family-Planning Programs for Teenagers on Adolescent Birth and Pregnancy Rates" and "Effects of Family-Planning Programs on Teenage Pregnancy—Replication and Extension," *Family Perspective* Fall 1986, pp. 154-195; and *Wall Street Journal*, 10/14/86.

25. Report of the U. S. House Select Committee on Children, Youth, and Families, *Teen Pregnancy: What Is Being Done? A State-By-State Look* (Washington, D.C.: Government Printing Office, 1986), p. 20. Updated data from "Trends: Adolescent Pregnancy, Abortion, and Childbearing," Family Life Information Exchange (Rockville, Md., May 1987), pp. 1-4.
26. Testimony cited in Peden and Glahe, eds., *The American Family*, p. 356.
27. Kasun, "Teenage Pregnancy: What Comparisons among States and Countries Show."
28. Phillips Cutright, "Illegitimacy in the United States: 1920-1968," in Robert Parke, Jr., and Charles F. Westoff, *Research Reports*, U. S. Commission of Population Growth and the American Future, vol. 1 (Washington, D.C.: Government Printing Office), p. 121.
29. Peden and Glahe, eds., *The American Family*, p. 358.
30. Jones, "Teenage Pregnancy in Developed Countries," pp. 53-62.
31. Olsen and Weed, "Effects of Family-Planning Programs," pp. 154, 173.
32. Louis Harris and Associates, *American Teens Speak: Sex, Myths, T.V. and Birth Control* (New York: Harris and Associates, 1986).
33. *Family Planning Perspective* (May/June 1981), p. 108, as cited in Peden and Glahe, eds., *The American Family*, p. 354.
34. Frederick S. Jaffe, testimony in hearings before the House Select Committee on Population, "Fertility and Conception in America," no. 13, pp. 537-550, as cited in Peden and Glahe, eds., *The American Family*, p. 354.
35. Melvin Zelnik and John F. Kantner, "Sexual Activity, Contraceptive Use and Pregnancy Among Metropolitan Area Teenagers, 1971-1979," *Family Planning Perspectives* (September/October 1980), pp. 230-237.
36. "Does Contraception Prevent Abortion," Human Life Center, 1983.
37. Frances Frech, "Update on Teen Pregnancies," *Heartbeat Quarterly* (Summer 1980).
38. U. S. House Select Committee on Children, Youth, and Families.
39. *Teenage Pregnancy: The Problem That Hasn't Gone Away*, p. 21, as cited in Peden and Glahe, eds., *The American Family*, p. 362.
40. Vito M. Logrillo, et al, *Effects of Induced Abortion on Subsequent Reproductive Function*, Final Report (New York State Department of Health, 4/18/80), p. 10, as cited in Peden and Glahe, eds., *The American Family*, p. 362.
41. *Teenage Pregnancy: The Problem That Hasn't Gone Away*, p. 5, as cited in Barrett Mosbacker, "Clinics, Children, and Control," in *School-Based Clinics* (Westchester, Ill.: Crossway, 1987), p. 65.
42. *The Knickerbocker Times*, Albany, New York, 12/6/63. As cited in Judie Brown, et al, *Stop School-Based Sex Clinics* (Stafford, Va.: American Life League, 1987) pp. 7-8.
43. *Family Practice News*, 12/15/77, as cited in Brown.
44. New York *Times*, 6/12/81, as cited in Brown.
45. A. Pietropinto, "A Survey on Contraception Analysis," *Medical Aspects of Human Sexuality*, May 1987, p. 147.
46. Frank Furstenberg, et al, *Teenage Sexuality, Pregnancy, and Childbearing* (Pittsburgh: U. of Pennsylvania Press, 1981).
47. Hayes, *Risking the Future*, p. 165.
48. Kingsley Davis, "The American Family, Relation to Demographic Change," in Robert Parke, Jr., and Charles F. Westoff, *Research Reports*, p. 253.

II. SCHOOL-BASED CLINICS FOR ADOLESCENTS

49. Mosbacker, in *School-Based Clinics*, p. 67.
50. Ibid.
51. See announcements for "Adolescence: Coming of Age in America," a conference held in Houston, Texas, 10/22-24/86.
52. Faye Wattleton, speech reprinted in the *Humanist* (July/August 1986), p. 7, as cited in Mosbacker, in *School-Based Clinics*, p. 66.
53. Douglas Kirby, *School-Based Health Clinics: An Emerging Approach to Improving Adolescent Health and Addressing Teenage Pregnancy*, Center for Population Options, April 1985, pp. 18-21, as cited in Mosbacker, in *School-Based Clinics*, pp. 67-68.
54. Ibid., pp. 7-8, as cited in Mosbacker, in *School-Based Clinics*, p. 71.
55. New York *Times*, 5/19/86.

56. See "Adolescents: Coming of Age" and California Alliance Concerned with School Aged Parents, Workshops on SBCs, 11/13-15/86.
57. Asta M. Kenney, "School-Based Clinics: A National Conference," *Family Planning Perspectives* (January/February 1986), p. 45.
58. Barrett Mosbacker, *Teen Pregnancy and School-Based Health Clinics* (Washington, D.C.: Family Research Council, August 1986), p. 6.
59. Laura Edwards, et al, "Adolescent Pregnancy Prevention Services in High School Clinics," *Family Planning Perspectives* (January/February 1980), pp. 311-314.
60. Kirby, *School-Based Health Clinics*, p. 14, as cited in Mosbacker, *School-Based Clinics*, p. 73.
61. Kenney, "School-Based Clinics: A National Conference," pp. 44-46.
62. Michael Schwartz, "Lies, Damned Lies, and Statistics," *American Education Report* (March 1986), p. 4, as cited in Mosbacker, *School-Based Clinics*, p. 73.
63. Marie Dietz, unpublished paper, "St. Paul In-School Sex Clinics," no date, as cited in Mosbacker, *School-Based Clinics*, p. 73.
64. Peden and Glahe, eds., *The American Family*, pp. 358-359.
65. Ibid., p. 359.
66. Jacqueline Kasun, "The Baltimore School Birth Control Study: A Comment," Humboldt State University, p. 1.
67. Ibid.
68. Ibid., p. 2.
69. Centers for Disease Control, *Teenage Pregnancy and Fertility Trends—United States 1976, 1980,* MMWR, 1985, p. 277, as cited in S. Dubose Ravenel, M.D., "American Teens and Birth Control: Commentary," *North Carolina Medical Journal* (November 1987), p. 607.
70. Kasun, "The Baltimore School Birth Control Study," pp. 2-3.
71. Tobin Demsko, "School-Based Health Clinics: A Look at the Johns Hopkins Study" (Washington, D.C.: Family Research Council), pp. 6-7.
72. Ibid., p. 8.
73. Ibid., pp. 5-6.
74. Mike Yorkey, "SBCs on the Move," *Focus on the Family* (October 1986), p. 4.
75. Ibid., pp. 4-5 and Chicago *Tribune*, 2/26/87.
76. *National Right to Life News*, 3/10/88.
77. Myron Lieberman, "Sex Education," *Journal of Family and Culture* (Winter 1986), p. 58.

III. COMPREHENSIVE SEX EDUCATION

78. Jacqueline Kasun, "The Truth About Sex Education," in Mosbacker, *School-Based Clinics*, p. 38.
79. Jones, "Teenage Pregnancy in Developed Countries," pp. 53-62.
80. "Not in the Public Interest: The Planned Parenthood Version of Sex Education" (Cincinnati: Couple to Couple League, 1981), p. 1.
81. Harris and Associates, *American Teens Speak*, p. 50.
82. Melvin Zelnik and Young J. Kim, "Sex Education and Its Association With Teenage Sexual Activity, Pregnancy, and Contraceptive Use," *Family Planning Perspective* (May/June 1982), p. 118.
83. Hayes, *Risking the Future*, p. 144.
84. William Marsiglio and Frank Mott, "The Impact of Sex Education on Sexual Activity, Contraceptive Use, and Premarital Pregnancy Among American Teenagers," *Family Planning Perspectives* (July/August 1986).
85. Harris and Associates, *American Teens Speak*, p. 50.
86. "AIDS Education Needs Assessment," conducted in December 1987 by the Council of Chief State School Officers and released 7/8/88. Reported in the *Education Reporter*, August 1988.
87. Julie Lapore, "A National Call to Action," *Emphasis*, Autumn 1987, p. 4.
88. Melvin Zelnik, et al, *Sex and Pregnancy in Adolescence* (Beverly Hills, Ca.: Sage Publications, 1981), p. 179, as cited in Peden and Glahe, eds., *The American Family*, p. 358.
89. Zelnik and Kim, "Sex Education and Its Association With Teenage Sexual Activity," pp. 117-126.

90. National Education Association, "What Parents Should Know About Sex Education in the Schools," as cited in Kasun, "The Truth About Sex Education," p. 35.

91. Douglas Kirby, "Sexuality Education: A More Realistic View of Its Effects," *Journal of School Health* (December 1985), p. 422, as cited in Mosbacker, *School-Based Clinics*, pp. 64-65.

92. San Antonio *Express News*, March 3, 1989.

93. Deborah Dawson, "The Effects of Sex Education on Adolescent Behavior," *Family Planning Perspectives* (July/August, 1986), p. 169.

94. Surgeon General's *Report on Acquired Immune Deficiency Syndrome* (October 1986), and joint statement issued by William Bennett and C. Everett Koop, 1/30/87.

95. Shirley Hartley, *Illegitimacy* (Berkeley: U. of California Press, 1975), as cited in Kasun, "The Truth About Sex Education," p. 35.

96. Bruno Bettelheim, interviewed by Elizabeth Hall, "Our Children Are Treated Like Idiots," *Psychology Today* (July 1981), pp. 28-44, as cited in Peden and Glahe, eds., *The American Family*, p. 357.

97. Marsiglio and Mott, "The Impact of Sex Education on Sexual Activity," p. 151.

98. Review of Peter R. Kilmann, et al, "Sex Education: A Review of Its Effects," *Archives of Sexual Behavior* 10 (no. 2, 1981), pp. 177-205, appearing in *Family Life Educator* Preview Issue (May 1982), p. 27, as cited in Kasun, "The State and Adolescent Sexual Behavior," p. 356.

99. Furstenberg, et al, *Teenage Sexuality, Pregnancy, and Childbearing.*

100. Sean O'Reilly, *Sex Education in the Schools* (Thaxton, Va.: Sun Life, 1978).

101. Melvin Anchell, "Psychoanalysis v. Sex Education," *National Review,* 6/20/86, p. 33.

102. Report of the U. S. House Select Committee on Children, Youth, and Families, *Teen Pregnancy: What Is Being Done?,* p. 386.

103. Jerome T. Y. Shen, "Adolescent Sexual Counseling," *Adolescent Sexuality* (May 1982), as cited in Judie Brown, et al, *Stop School-Based Sex Clinics* (Stafford, Va.: American Life League, 1987).

104. Josh McDowell, *Adolescent Sexuality Research Digest* (Dallas: Josh McDowell Ministries, n.d.), p. 10.

105. Norman B. Ryder, "Contraceptive Failure in the United States," *Family Planning Perspective* (Summer 1973), pp. 133-142.

106. Zelnik and Kantner, "Contraceptive Patterns," p. 138 and Table 8.

107. William Grady, et al, "Contraceptive Failure in the United States—Estimates from the 1982 National Survey of Family Growth," *Family Planning Perspective* (September/October 1986), pp. 200-207.

108. Martin Fisher, et al, "Comparative Analysis of the Effectiveness of the Diaphragm and Birth Control Pill During the First Year of Use Among Suburban Adolescents," *Journal of Adolescent Health Care* (September 1987), pp. 393, 395.

109. Zelnik and Kantner, "Sexual Activity, Contraceptive Use, and Pregnancy," p. 236.

110. Fisher, et al, "Comparative Analysis," p. 397.

111. FDA package insert, as cited in Brown, et al, *Stop School-Based Sex Clinics.*

112. Ibid.

113. *U.S. News and World Report,* 6/2/86.

114. Sol Gordon, et al, *Raising a Child Conservatively in a Sexually Permissive World* (New York: Simon and Schuster, 1983), p. 166, as cited in McDowell, *Adolescent Sexuality Research Digest*, p. 14.

115. "Sexually Active Teens May Lead Age Groups in Chlamydia Rate," *OB-GYN News*, 1/1-14/86.

116. S. L. Barron, "Sexual Activity in Girls Under 16 Years of Age," *British Journal of Obstetrics and Gynecology,* 1986, vol. 93, p. 787.

117. W. Cates, Jr. and J. L. Rauh, "Adolescents and Sexually Transmitted Diseases: An Expanding Problem," *Journal of Adolescent Health Care,* vol. 6, no. 4, pp. 257-260.

118. *Pediatric News* (August 1988), p. 31.

119. A. Eugene Washington, et al, "Pelvic Inflammatory Disease and Its Sequelae in Adolescents," *Journal of Adolescent Health Care* (July 1985), pp. 298-309.

120. U. S. Department of Education, "Will 'Safe Sex' Education Effectively Combat AIDS?," informal paper, 1/22/88.

121. San Antonio *Express*, 6/18/88.

122. *USA Today,* 9/18/87.

123. Margaret A. Fischl, et al, "Evaluation of Heterosexual Partners, Children and Household Contacts of Adults With AIDS," *Journal of the American Medical Association* 257:640 (1987).

124. Dr. Theresa Crenshaw, testimony before the U. S. House Select Committee on Children, Youth, and Families, 6/18/87.

125. Seattle *Times,* 8/10/88.

126. U. S. Department of Education, "Will 'Safe Sex' Education Effectively Combat AIDS?" and "AIDS and the Education of Our Children: Guide for Parents and Teachers," October 1987.

127. "Update on Condoms—Products, Protection, Promotion," *Population Reports* (September/ October 1982), pp. H121-122.

128. Bruce Voeller and Malcolm Potts, *British Medical Journal* (October 1985), p. 1196.

129. William Grady, et al, "Contraceptive Failure in the United States," pp. 203, 204, 207.

130. Lode Wigersma and Ron Oud, "Safety and Acceptability of Condoms for Use by Homosexual Men as a Prophylactic Against Transmission of HIV During Anogenital Sexual Intercourse," *British Medical Journal* (7/11/87), p. 94, and correspondence of Dr. Wigersma (10/14/87), as cited in U. S. Department of Education, "Will 'Safe Sex' Education Effectively Combat AIDS?," pp. 11, 25.

131. *Insight* (6/22/87), p. 7.

132. FDA, *Compliance Policy Guidelines,* chapter 24, guide 7124. (4/10/87), p. 1.

133. *FDA Medical Devices Bulletin* (September 1987), p. 1.

134. Ronald O. Valdiserri, et al, "Condom Use in a Cohort of Gay and Bisexual Men," *Third International Conference on AIDS,* Washington, D.C., 6/1-5/87, *Abstracts Volume,* p. 213.

135. Joint statement of Bennett and Koop and James J. Goedert, "What Is Safe Sex? Suggested Standards Linked to Testing for Human Immunodeficiency Virus," *New England Journal of Medicine* (5/21/87), pp. 1339-1341.

136. U. S. House Select Committee on Children, Youth, and Families, *Teen Pregnancy: What Can Be Done?,* p. 20.

137. Harris and Associates, *American Teens Speak,* p. 50. See, e.g., the newsletter for teens *Birth Control Confidential* (Summer 1987), p. 2, in which early abortions are promoted.

138. Willard Cates, et al, "The Risks Associated with Teenage Abortion," *The New England Journal of Medicine* (9/15/83), pp. 621-624.

139. Willard Cates, "Legal Abortion: The Public Health Record," *Science* (3/26/82), pp. 1586-1590.

140. "Ectopic Pregnancies—United States, 1970-1980," *Journal of the American Medical Association* (5/11/84), p. 223.

141. Polly A. Marchbanks, et al, "Risk Factors for Ectopic Pregnancy," *Journal of the American Medical Association* (3/25/88), pp. 1823-1827.

142. Cates, "Legal Abortion."

143. Kenneth McAll and William Wilson, "Ritual Mourning for Unresolved Grief After Abortion," *Southern Medical Journal* (July 1987), pp. 817-821.

144. John S. Lyons, et al, "Research on the Psychosocial Impact of Abortion: A Systematic Review of the Literature of 1966 to 1985," in Gerald P. Regier, ed., *Values and Public Policy* (Washington, D.C.: Family Research Council of America, 1988), pp. 77-89.

145. Kasun, "The Truth About Sex Education," pp. 29-30.

146. Alfred De Maris and Gerald R. Leslie, "Cohabitation With the Future Spouse: Its Influence Upon Marital Satisfaction and Communication," *Journal of Marriage and the Family* (February 1984), pp. 77-84, and *Religion Report,* 6/10/88.

147. See, e.g., California State Department of Education, *Education for Human Sexuality: A Resource Book and Instructional Guide to Sex Education for Kindergarten Through Grade Twelve* (1979).

148. Jones, et al, "Teenage Pregnancy in Developed Countries," pp. 53-62.

149. Koop statement, October 1986.

150. Hayes, *Risking the Future,* p. 144.

151. Centers for Disease Control, "AIDS Weekly Surveillance Report," 10/26/87, p. 5.

152. Centers for Disease Control, "AIDS Weekly Surveillance Report," 9/14/87.

153. Melvin Anchell, "Psychoanalysis v. Sex Education," p. 33.

154. Sean O'Reilly, *Sex Education in the Schools.*

155. Ibid.

156. Ibid.

157. Peden and Glahe, eds., *The American Family*, p. 357.
158. David Elkind, *The Hurried Child* (Reading, Mass.: Addison-Wesley, 1981), pp. 60-61.
159. Wanda Franz, "Adolescent Cognitive Abilities and Implications for Sexual Decision Making," paper presented at Celebrate the Family Third Eastern Symposium, Pennsylvania State University, 3/24/87, pp. 1, 3.
160. Ibid., pp. 6-7.
161. Ibid., pp. 7-8.
162. Ibid., pp. 10-12.
163. Ibid., pp. 18-19.
164. Ibid., p. 14; L. Kohlberg, "Development of Moral Character and Moral Ideology," *Review of Child Development Research* (New York: Sage Foundation, 1964); and L. Kohlberg, "Stage and Sequence: The Cognitive-Developmental Approach to Socialization," in D. A. Goslin, ed., *Handbook of Socialization Theory and Research* (Chicago: Rand McNally, 1969). NOTE: Kohlberg's stages of moral reasoning have limitations and should not serve as an exclusive basis from which to build a moral foundation. See discussion of Kohlberg in William Coulson, Ph.D., "Focus: Classroom Courses Promote Drugs and Sex," *The Education Reporter*, June 1988.
165. Franz, "Adolescent Cognitive Abilities," p. 14.
166. Ibid.
167. William Bennett, "Sex and the Education of Our Children," in Mosbacker, *School-Based Clinics*, p. 162.
168. Ibid., p. 161.

IV. INFLUENCING TODAY'S YOUTH

169. U. S. House Select Committee on Children, Youth, and Families, *Teen Pregnancy: What Can Be Done?*, p. 386.
170. Johnston Company synthesis of 18 studies for youth and values-oriented clients, 1954-80, as cited in McDowell, *Adolescent Sexuality Research Digest*, p. 25.
171. Adapted from W. Baldwin, "Adolescent Pregnancy and Childbearing—Growing Concern for Americans," *Population Bulletin* 31:1-36, updated reprint, as cited in McDowell, *Adolescent Sexuality Research Digest*, pp. 16-17. Updated data from "Trends: Adolescent Pregnancy, Abortion, and Childbearing," Family Life Information Exchange (Rockville, Md., May 1987), pp. 1-4.
172. Terrance Olson, Christopher M. Wallace, and Brent C. Miller, "Primary Prevention of Adolescent Pregnancy: Promoting Family Involvement Through a School Curriculum," *Journal of Primary Prevention* (Winter 1984), p. 81.
173. Ibid., pp. 81-82.
174. Melvin Zelnik and John F. Kantner, "Contraceptive Pattern and Premarital Pregnancy Among Women Aged 15-19 in 1976," *Family Planning Perspectives* (May/June 1978), p. 140, Table 3.
175. Pittsburgh *Courier*, 7/21/84.
176. Leon Dash, "At Risk: Chronicles of Teen-Age Pregnancy," Washington *Post*, 1/26-31/86.
177. Olson, Wallace, and Miller, "Primary Prevention of Adolescent Pregnancy," p. 82.
178. S. M. Fisher and K. R. Scharf, "Teenage Pregnancy: An Anthropological, Sociological, and Psychological Overview," *Adolescent Reactions to Divorce*, 1980.
179. Olson, Wallace, and Miller, "Primary Prevention of Adolescent Pregnancy," pp. 83-84.
180. Ibid., p. 85.
181. Ibid., pp. 85-86.
182. Terrance Olson and Christopher Wallace, "A Sampler of AANCHOR" (Provo, Utah: Brigham Young U.), pp. 34-35.
183. Ibid., p. 37.
184. Ibid., p. 38.
185. Ibid., p. 39.

186. U. S. Department of Health and Human Services, fact sheet, "Adolescent Pregnancy and Childbearing," p. 3; Leslie Jane Nonkin, *I Wish My Parents Understood* (New York: Penguin, 1985), p. 67; and Merton P. Strommen and Irene A. Strommen, *Five Cries of Parents* (San Francisco: Harper & Row, 1985), p. 72.

187. Zelnik and Kantner, "Sexual Activity, Contraceptive Use, and Pregnancy," pp. 230-237.

188. B. C. Miller, "Teenage Pregnancy: A Comparison of Certain Characteristics Among Utah Youth," report for the Utah State Office of Education (1981); Melvin Zelnik and John F. Kantner, unpublished tabulations from the National Longitudinal Survey of Youth, 1983, cited in Mosbacker, *Teenage Pregnancy*, p. 8; U. S. House Select Committee on Children, Youth, and Families, *Teen Pregnancy: What Can Be Done?*, p. 395; and Hayes, *Risking the Future*, pp. 54-55.

189. Harris and Associates, *American Teens Speak*, pp. 18, 24.

190. Melvin Zelnik and John F. Kantner, "Sexual and Contraceptive Experience of Unmarried Women in the United States, 1976 and 1971," *Family Planning Perspective* 9:2, pp. 55-71 and Table 2.

191. James F. Ford and Michael Schwartz, "Birth Control for Teenagers: Diagram for Disaster," *Linacre Quarterly* (February 1979), p. 76.

V. ABSTINENCE EDUCATION

192. Allan Carlson, "Pregnant Teenagers and Moral Civil War," in Mosbacker, *School-Based Clinics*, p. 16.

193. *Time*, 4/9/84.

194. Alexandra Mark and Vernon H. Mark, *Medical World News* (4/8/85), p. 156.

195. Office of Population Affairs, *The Adolescent Family Life Demonstration Projects*, pp. i-ii.

196. Coleen Kelly Mast, *Implementation Guide: Sex Respect Educational Program* (Bradley, Ill.: Respect, Inc., 1987), p. 3, and "Memorandum for the Secretary of Health and Human Services" (Washington, D.C.: The White House, Office of the Press Secretary), 9/8/88.

197. Ibid.

198. Bennett, "Sex and the Education of Our Children," p. 158.

199. Bennett and Koop, joint statement, 1/30/87.

200. Mast, *Implementation Guide*.

201. James H. Ford, "Rx: Adolescent Abstinence," adopted by the California Medical Association and the American Medical Association in 1984.

202. "Adolescent Abstinence Resolution," adopted by the 1987 Chapter Forum and reported in the *AAP News* (November 1987), p. 11, resolution #63.

203. 85th General Assembly, State of Illinois, 1987 and 1988, House Bill 1225.

204. Indiana First Regular Session 105th General Assembly, Senate Enrolled Act no. 72; Indiana Second Regular Session 105th General Assembly, House Enrolled Act no. 1067.

205. State of Washington, Senate Bill 6221. Passed March 1988. Portions of this omnibus bill do not meet the standards recommended in this report. The bill should be scrutinized carefully.

206. Florida 1988 Committee Substitute H.B. 1519. Portions of this omnibus bill do not meet the standards outlined in this report and should be scrutinized carefully.

207. California Senate Bill 2394. Passed August 1988.

208. General Assembly Commonwealth of Kentucky, House Bill 345. Signed into law 4/1/88. There is a loophole in the law's language, however, that could allow the wrong type of education to be used.

209. The Missouri Task Force on Unwed Adolescent Sexual Activity and Pregnancy, final report, *A Time to Speak. . A Time to Act*, December 1987.

210. Linda Moore, Assistant to California State Senator Newton Russell. Interview with Dinah Richard, February 24, 1989.

211. Texas House Bills 226, 304, 329, and 493 were defeated in 1986. In Pennsylvania, Peg Luksik and the Pennsylvania Parents' Commission have helped defeat a series of bills that would have mandated the wrong type of education.

212. *Education Reporter*, January 1988.

213. Los Angeles *Times*, March 9, 1986.

214. St. Louis *Globe-Democrat,* 10/25-26/86.

215. U. S. Department of Education, "Will 'Safe Sex Education' Effectively Combat AIDS?"

216. *Liberty Report,* September 1987.

217. Chicago *Tribune,* 4/22/86.

218. Supreme Court of the United States, Bowen v. Kendrick, nos. 87-253, 87-431, 87-462, and 87-775. 6/29/88.

219. Hayes, *Risking the Future,* pp. 54-55.

220. Bennett, "Sex and the Education of Our Children," in Mosbacker, *School-Based Clinics,* p. 164.

221. Marion Howard, "Postponing Sexual Involvement Among Adolescents," *Journal of Adolescent Health Care* (July 1985), pp. 271-277.

222. Murray L. Vincent, et al, "Reducing Adolescent Pregnancy Through School and Community Based Education," *Journal of the American Medical Association* (6/26/87), pp. 3382-3388.

223. Yorkey, "SBCs on the Move" and Chicago *Tribune,* 2/26/87.

224. Kurt Back, as cited in Terrance Olson, "Adolescent Pregnancy and Abstinence: How Far Have We Come," Brigham Young University, unpublished speech on the AANCHOR project, p. 2.

225. *U.S. News and World Report,* 6/30/86, as cited in McDowell, *Adolescent Sexuality Research Digest.*

226. UPI release, 9/12/87.

227. Bennett, "Sex and the Education of Our Children," p. 164.

228. Philadelphia *Inquirer,* 7/10/86.

229. Harris and Associates, *American Teens Speak,* p. 71.

230. Washington *Post,* 6/6/83.

231. Bennett, "Sex and the Education of Our Children," p. 162.

232. *Young Adolescents and Their Parents* (Minneapolis: Search Institute, 1984).

233. Bennett, "Sex and the Education of Our Children," pp. 167-168.

234. Franz, "Adolescent Cognitive Abilities," pp. 20-21.

235. Family Research Council, fact sheet, "Values-Based Sex Education Resources," pp. 1-2.

236. Olson and Wallace, "A Sampler of AANCHOR," p. 32.

237. Ibid., p. 33.

238. Los Angeles *Times,* 10/17/86.

239. Search Institute, *Human Sexuality: Values and Choices.*

240. Marion Howard, et al, *Postponing Sexual Involvement* (Atlanta: Emory/Grady Teen Services, Grady Memorial Hospital).

241. Vincent, et al, "Reducing Adolescent Pregnancy Through School and Community Based Education," pp. 3382-88.

242. Olson, "Adolescent Pregnancy and Abstinence," unpublished speech, pp. 5-6.

243. Harris and Associates, *American Teens Speak,* p. 53. Louis Harris and Associates, "The Relationships Between Sexual Activity and Sex Education." And telephone interview between Dinah Richard and Jacqueline Kasun, January 5, 1989. See also, Jacqueline Kasun, "Sex Education: The Hidden Agenda," *The World and I,* September 1989, pp. 494-495.

244. See, for example, the Houston Independent School District's Family Life/Health Education program for sixth graders, "Information for the Teacher, Methods of Contraception," 6W8-27.194. Planned Parenthood helped put together the Houston family life program.

245. Office of Population Affairs, *The Adolescent Family Life Demonstration Projects,* pp. 242-246.

246. Olson and Wallace, "A Sampler of AANCHOR," p. 35.

247. *The Teen-Aid Family Life Education Project.* An Evaluation Report prepared for the Office of Adolescent Pregnancy Program (OAPP) by the Institute for Research and Evaluation, December 28, 1988. Stan E. Weed, Joseph A. Olsen, and Raja Tanas, Project Evaluators.

248. Dinah Richard telephone interview with Nancy Hughes, School Nurse, Lamar Junior High School, Lamar, Missouri, April 1989.

249. UPI release, 1/12/88, and studies compiled by Project Respect for the second-year pilot program. Similar results are available for the third year.

250. Ibid.

251. Los Angeles *Times,* 3/6/86.

252. Joe DeDiminicantanio to LeAnna Benn, 10/2/87.

253. Ibid.

254. "Teen Choice Project Evaluation: Interim Evaluation Report," draft, 7/18/88; Teen Choice press release, 8/1/88; letter from Martha Long, assistant director of Teen Choice, to Dinah Richard, 7/16/88.

255. Bennett and Koop, joint statement, 1/30/87.

256. Mast, *Implementation Guide*, p. 10.

VI. PARENTAL INVOLVEMENT

257. U. S. House Select Committee on Children, Youth, and Families, *Teen Pregnancy: What Can Be Done?*, p. 387.

258. Office of Population Affairs, *The Adolescent Family Life Demonstration Projects*, p. 287.

259. Orrin Hatch amendment, The Education Amendment of 1978, Public Law 95-561, 11/1/78.

260. Dinah Richard telephone interview with Joe DeDiminicantanio, Principal of San Marcos Junior High School, San Marcos, California, April 1989.

261. London *Daily Telegraph*, 9/27/85.

262. U. S. House Select Committee on Children, Youth and Families, *Teen Pregnancy: What Can Be Done?*, pp. 387, 380.

263. London *Daily Telegraph*, 9/27/85.

264. Olson and Wallace, "A Sampler of AANCHOR," p. 35.

265. Educational Guidance Institute, Inc., "Parents and Teens Learn to Communicate About Sexual Values in New Family Life Education Program," press release, February 22, 1989.

266. Fertility Appreciation for Families, "Program Description: Wonder of Love and Life, Demonstration Project," summary report.

267. Ibid.

268. Letter from Anne Nesbit, author and director of LAMO, to Dinah Richard, 7/19/87.

APPENDIX A
ARTICLES AND BOOKS ON CONTEMPORARY APPROACHES
AND THE NEED FOR INNOVATIVE EDUCATION

Anchell, Melvin. "Psychoanalysis v. Sex Education," *National Review,* 6/20/86.

Brown, Judie, et al. *Stop School-Based Sex Clinics.* Stafford, Virginia: American Life League, 1987.

Echaniz, Judith. *When Schools Teach Sex . . A Handbook for Evaluating Your School's Sex Education Program.* Rochester, New York: Family-Life Culture and Education Council, Free Congress Research & Education Foundation, 1982.

Ford, James H., and Michael Schwartz. "Birth Control for Teenagers: Diagram for Disaster, *Linacre Quarterly,* February 1979, pp. 71-81.

Ford, James H. "Rx: Adolescent Abstinence." Reprinted by the American Life League.

Franz, Wanda. "Adolescent Cognitive Abilities and Implications for Sexual Decision Making." Paper presented at Celebrate the Family Third Eastern Symposium, Pennsylvania State University, 3/24/87.

Kasun, Jacqueline. "The State and Adolescent Sexual Behavior," in Joseph R. Peden and Fred R. Glahe, eds., *The American Family and the State.* San Francisco: Pacific Research Institute for Public Policy, 1986.

Marshall, Robert. *School Birth Control, New Promise or Old Problem?* Stafford, Virginia: American Life League, 1986.

Mast, Coleen. *Implementation Guide.* Bradley, Illinois: Respect, Inc., 1987.

McDowell, Josh. "Action Packet." Dallas: Josh McDowell Ministries, 1987.

McDowell, Josh. *Adolescent Sexuality Research Digest.* Dallas: Josh McDowell Ministries, 1987.

Missouri Task Force on Unwed Adolescent Sexual Activity and Pregnancy, "A Time to Speak...A Time to Act." December 1987.

Mosbacker, Barrett. *Teen Pregnancy and School-Based Health Clinics.* Washington, D.C.: Family Research Council, 1986.

Mosbacker, Barrett. *School-Based Clinics.* Westchester, Illinois: Crossway, 1987.

Olsen, Joseph, and Stan Weed. "Effects of Family Planning Programs for Teenagers on Adolescent Birth and Pregnancy Rates" and "Effects of Family Planning Programs on Teenage Pregnancy—Replication and Extension," *Family Perspective,* Brigham Young University, vol. 20, no. 3, 1986, pp. 153-195. Also reprinted by the Family Research Council of America.

Olson, Terrance, et al. "Primary Prevention of Adolescent Pregnancy: Promoting Family Involvement Through a School Curriculum,"

O'Reilly, Sean. *Sex Education in the Schools.* Thaxton, Virginia: Sun Life, 1978.

Journal of Primary Prevention, Winter 1984, pp. 75-91.

Schwartz, Michael, and James Ford. "Family Planning Clinics: Cure or Cause of Teenage Pregnancy?" *Linacre Quarterly,* May 1982, pp. 143-164.

Socia, Pat. *Teaching True Abstinence Education.* Golf, Illinois: Project Respect, 1989.

U. S. House Select Committee on Children, Youth, and Families. *Teen Pregnancy: What Is Being Done? A State-By-State Look.* Washington, D.C.: Government Printing Office, 1986, pp. 373-397.

Weed, Stan. "Current Patterns and Programs for Teenage Pregnancy Prevention: A Summary for Policy Makers," Washington, D.C.: Government Printing Office, 1989.

Weed, Stan, and Joseph Olsen. "Policy and Program Considerations for Teenage Pregnancy Prevention: A Summary for Policy Makers," *Family Perspective,* Brigham Young University, Vol. 22, No. 3, 1989, pp. 235-252.

Yorkey, Mike. "SBCs on the Move," *Focus on the Family,* October 1986, pp. 2-5.

APPENDIX B
AUDIOVISUAL RESOURCES FOR ADULTS ON THE TEENAGE SEXUALITY CRISIS AND EVALUATION OF THE CONTRACEPTIVE APPROACH

Abstinence Education Works...Here's How!
A videotape of Mike Long of Project Respect, discussing the importance and effectiveness of abstinence education. Available from Project Respect, Committee on the Status of Women, Box 97, Golf, IL 60029-0097, (312) 729-3298.

A Critical Look at Planned Parenthood
Two slide presentations that take a critical look at Planned Parenthood. Available from Vital Signs, P.O. Box 1279, Tryon, NC 28782, (704) 859-5392.

How to Stop School-Based Sex Clinics
A video featuring twenty national leaders who oppose school-based clinics. Available from American Life League, Box 1350, Stafford, VA 22554, (703) 659-4171.

Myths of Sex Education
A 45-minute video in which Josh McDowell examines the secular agenda as it relates to sex education, exposing common myths about comprehensive sex instruction. Available from Josh McDowell Ministries, Box 1000, Dallas, TX 75221, (214) 907-1000.

New Perspectives in Education
A video of a full-day workshop by Dr. William Coulsen, former researcher for Carl Rogers and Abraham Maslow. Dr. Coulsen describes the detrimental effects that humanist psychology have had on our educational system. NOTE: The production values of the video are not highest quality, Dr. Coulsen's presentation is very stimulating. Available through People for Responsible Education, 420 N. Seventh St., Barron, WI 54812.

Project Sex Respect
A videotape in which LeAnna Benn of Teen-Aid and Coleen Mast of Respect, Inc. give overviews of their public school abstinence curricula. Available from Womanity, 1700 Oak Park Blvd, Room C-4, Pleasant Hill, CA 94523, (415) 943-6424.

Promo Video: Sex Respect
Coleen Mast talks about the need for abstinence education in the schools. Available from Respect, Inc., P.O. Box 349, Bradley, IL 60915-0349, (815) 932-8389.

School-Based Health Clinics
A videotape of two talks given at a national conference. In the first part, Stan Weed discusses his statistical research showing the failure of teen family planning services. In the second part, Helen Blackwell gives practical advice for opposing SBCs. Available from Concerned Women for America, 370 L'Enfant Promenade SW, Suite 800, Washington, DC 20024, (800) 458-8797.

School Sex Clinics
A videotape exposing the danger of school-based clinics. Available from Womanity, 1700 Oak Park Blvd, Room C-4, Pleasant Hill, CA 94523, (415) 943-6424.

Where Youth Are Today
A video talking about the teenage sexuality crisis from a Christian perspective. Available from Word, Inc., P.O. Box 2518, Waco, TX 76702, (817) 772-7650.

Why Wait? Preview Tape
Contains interviews with various national leaders who are calling for a morally based abstinence approach to the teenage sexuality crisis. From a Christian perspective. Also comes with the eight-part video series, *How to Help Your Child Say 'No' to Sexual Pressure*. Available from Josh McDowell Ministries, Box 1000, Dallas, TX 75221, (214) 907-1000.

APPENDIX C
APPROPRIATE CURRICULA FOR PUBLIC SCHOOLS

AANCHOR
A curriculum for junior or senior high school students in public schools. Designed to help teens learn how to live responsible lives by developing an understanding of and appreciation for premarital abstinence. Family oriented. Available from Dr. Terrance Olson, Department of Family Science, Brigham Young University, Provo, UT 84602, (801) 378-2069.

Facing Reality
A new high school curriculum by Project Respect, Box 97, Golf, IL 60029, (312) 729-3298.

Family Values and Sex Education
For public junior high schools. Focuses on how to live wise and happy lives that help young people avoid crises. Offers positive ways to say no. Available from Focus on the Family Publishing, Pomona, CA, 91799, (714) 620-8500.

Learning About Myself and Others (LAMO)
A program designed for children in grades one through six. Presented from a traditional perspective with an emphasis on premarital abstinence, traditional family, and marriage. Requires that parents attend along with children. Available from Anne Nesbit, P.R. #48 Orchard Circle, Pittsfield, MA 01201, (413) 698-2688.

Me, My World, My Future
A middle school program that stresses the postponement of immediate gratification in exchange for future goals in the areas of sexual activity, drugs, alcohol, and tobacco. A fifteen-unit program. Available from Teen-Aid, N. 1330 Calispel, Spokane, WA 99201, (509) 466-8679.

Sex and Self-Respect
A two- to five-day video-based curriculum for students aged 12-15 and their parents. Three tapes are provided: (1) A 24-minute tape for students which contains six scenarios dramatizing the psychological and physical advantages of premarital abstinence. High-quality acting and very captivating to teens. (2) A parental preview tape, containing the same content of the student tape, plus an introduction for parents and teachers. (3) A medical facts tape which gives information about sexually transmitted diseases, abortion, and other problems associated with teenage premarital sex. A teacher's guide accompanies the videos. Written by Dr. Paul Vitz, Department of Psychology, New York University, along with producer John Marler. Available from Character Curriculum, Inc., 112 E. Church St., Cuero, TX 77954, (800) 544-0760.

Sex Respect: The Option of True Sexual Freedom
A morally based abstinence curriculum consisting of three separate workbooks: one for teens, one for teachers, and one for parents. A three-week program for junior or senior high. Available from either Respect, Inc., P.O. Box 349, Bradley, IL 60915, (815) 932-8389, or Project Respect, Committee on the Status of Women, Box 97, Golf, IL 60029, (312) 729-3298. (Both Respect, Incorporated and Project Respect have also developed separate new high school curricula.)

Sexuality, Commitment, and Family
A three-week, morally based program for public high schools. Available from Teen-Aid, Inc., N. 1330 Calispel, Spokane, WA 99201, (509) 466-8679.

You Are Unique
A program requiring two or three 45-minute sessions dealing with individuality, gender differences, pressure to have sex, the freedoms of chastity and other topics. Available from Sex and Family Education, 1608—13th Ave. South, Birmingham, AL 35205, (205) 939-0302.

APPENDIX D
APPROPRIATE CURRICULA FOR CHURCHES
AND COMMUNITY GROUPS

Concordia Sex Education Series
A six-part series with books, filmstrips, and audio cassette tapes designed for elementary through secondary school. Presented from a Christian perspective. Available from Concordia Publishing House, 3558 S. Jefferson, St. Louis, MO 63118-3968, (800) 325-3040.

God Made You Unique
This series adds Scripture to the *You Are Unique* curriculum listed in Appendix C. Available from Sex and Family Education, 1608—13th Ave. South, Birmingham, AL 35205, (205) 939-0302.

Love and Life
A series developed by Coleen Mast, author of Sex Respect. Intended for private and Catholic schools. Available from Ignatius Press, 15 Oakland Avenue, Harrison, NY 10528, (914) 835-4216.

No—The Positive Answer
A four-part video series with an accompanying curriculum guide. Available in Christian and public school versions from Why Wait?, Josh McDowell Ministries, Box 1000, Dallas, TX 75221, (214) 907-1000.

APPENDIX E
PARENT TRAINING

Fertility Appreciation for Families

A family-centered curriculum. Two four-hour sessions, one for parents of children to age fourteen, and one for parents and their kids ages eleven to eighteen. The parent-teen curriculum uses slides and films. Available from Family of the Americas, 1150 Lovers Lane, Mandeville, LA 71448, (504) 626-7724.

How to Help Your Child Say "No" to Sexual Pressure

An eight-part video series for parents of teens and preteens. Designed to help parents become more effective as the primary educators of their children. Includes a leader's guide. Presented from a Christian perspective. Available from Josh McDowell Ministries, Box 1000, Dallas, Texas 75221, (214) 907-1000.

Let's Talk About Love & Sex

A videotape intended for home viewing by children and parents together. Covers general issues of sexuality and is designed to promote parent-teen discussion. Comes with a discussion manual. Available from Why Wait?, Josh McDowell Ministries, Box 1000, Dallas, TX 75221, (214) 907-1000.

A Parent's Guide: Teaching Responsible Sexual Behavior

A parent-training workshop that helps parents become the primary educators of their children. Five two-hour sessions. Available from Teen-Aid, N. 1330 Calispel, Spokane, WA 99201, (509) 466-8679.

APPENDIX F
FILMS FOR TEENS

Chastity Challenge
A videotape, from a Christian perspective, of Coleen Mast giving a presentation to teens. Two thirty-minute segments. Available from Respect, Inc., P.O. Box 349, Bradley, IL 60915, (815) 932-8389.

Control: It's Your Life
A film which targets the black teen with a dramatic presentation that covers the attitudes, options, and issues of sexuality. Encourages sound decision making and restraint. Available from New Dimension Films, 85895 Lorane Highway, Eugene, OR 97405, (503) 484-7125.

*Dating Movie**
A video for high school students that uses humor and drama to help young people understand love and premarital abstinence. From a Christian perspective. Available from Concordia Publishing, 3558 S. Jefferson, St. Louis, MO 63118-3968, (800) 325-3040.

Everyone Is Not Doing It
A video for high school students refuting the belief that all teens are "doing it." Emphasizes abstinence. Available from Project Respect, Box 97, Golf, IL 60029, (312) 729-3298.

*How to Handle the Pressure Lines**
A 30-minute video in which practical steps are given for resisting sexual pressure, plus advice on how to set positive dating standards. Available from Josh McDowell Ministries, Box 1000, Dallas, TX 75221, (214) 907-1000.

How to Know You're in Love
A film that shows a counseling session with a young couple. On free loan to public schools. Available from Gospel Films, Box 455, Muskegon, MI 49443, (800) 253-0413.

If You Want to Dance
An upbeat film showing the lives of two teenage girls who become pregnant and the consequences of premarital sex. Available from New Dimension Films, 85895 Lorane Highway, Eugene, OR 97405, (503) 484-7125.

Just Wait
A video for public schools containing interviews with teens discussing their views on sexuality. Builds the case for premarital abstinence. Available from Womanity, 1700 Oak Park Blvd., Room C-4, Pleasant Hill, CA 94523, (415) 943-6424.

*Let's Talk About Love and Sex**
A videotape intended for home viewing by children and parents together. Covers general issues of sexuality and is designed to prompt parent-teen discussion. Comes with a discussion manual. Available from Why Wait?, Josh McDowell Ministries, Box 1000, Dallas, TX 75221, (214) 907-1000.

Live, Laugh, Love*

A five-film series for teenagers. Accompanied by a curriculum guide for teachers. Contains Christian insights but has also been used widely in public schools. Available on free loan to public schools. Available from Gospel Films, Box 455, Muskegon, Michigan 49443, (800) 253-0413.

Love Waits*

A video featuring music and comments about abstinence in sexual relationships. Available from Christian Action Council, 701 W. Broad St., Suite 405, Falls Church, VA 22046, (703) 237-2100.

No Alibis

A 38-minute video for teens. Dramatizes the lives of two teenage girls faced with unplanned pregnancies. Available from Bridgestone Productions, 1991 Village Parkway, Suite 190, Encinitas, CA 92024, (619) 943-9200 or NRL Educational Trust, 419 Seventh St., NW, Suite 500, Washington, DC 20004, (202) 626-8800.

No—The Positive Answer*

A four-part video series with an accompanying curriculum guide. Designed for church use. Available from Why Wait?, Josh McDowell Ministries, Box 1000, Dallas, TX 75221, (214) 907-1000.

River of Fire

A film and video dealing with the life of a couple and the decision to wait. Discusses teenage sexuality, pregnancy, and STD. Available from New Dimension Films, 85895 Lorane Highway, Eugene, OR 97405, (503) 484-7125.

Safe Sex

A video for high schoolers on the choices teens face in dealing with the lies of "safe sex." Available from Gospel Films Inc., P.O. Box 455, Muskegon, MI 59443, (616) 773-3361.

Saving Sex for Marriage

A 15-minute video featuring young people's candid remarks about sex superimposed over scenes of a wedding. Available from Womanity Publications, 1700 Oak Park Blvd., Room C-4, Pleasant Hill, CA 94523, (415) 943-6424.

Sex and Self-Respect

A 24-minute video containing six scenarios in which teens dramatize the psychological and physical advantages of premarital abstinence. High-quality acting and very captivating to a teenage audience. This tape is one of three tapes described in the curriculum with the same title in Appendix C, Appropriate Curricula for Public Schools. Available from Character Curriculum, Inc., 112 E. Church St., Cuero, TX 77954, (800) 544-0760.

The Sexual Puzzle

A video for teenagers that talks about the conflicts they face and why they should abstain from sex. Comes in public school and Christian versions. Available from Josh McDowell Ministries, Box 1000, Dallas, TX 75221, (214) 907-1000.

Springtime of Your Life

A slide and audiocassette tape program covering the reasons for premarital abstinence. Available from Couple to Couple League, Box 11084, Cincinnati, OH 45211, (513) 661-7612.

Straight Talk About Love, Sex, and Dating*

A five-film series dealing with adolescent sexuality. Presented from a Christian perspective. Rental only. Available from Shepherd Ministries, 8006 Steven St., Irving, TX 75062, (214) 570-7599.

They Lied to Us*

A film with interviews of teenagers. From a Christian perspective. Rental only. Available from Word, Inc., P.O. Box 2518, Waco, TX 76702, (817) 772-7650.

Why Wait?

A video of a classroom discussion of teen sexuality. Available from Teen-Aid, N. 1330 Calispel, Spokane, WA 99201, (509) 466-8679.

Wounded Lovers*

A 36-minute video in which teenagers tell the real stories of how they became pregnant and the consequences of premarital sex. Christian insights; very moving accounts. Includes a 20-page workbook. Available from Living Parables, P.O. Box 187, Loomis, CA 95650, (800) 223-4826, in California (916) 888-7682.

Young Fathers*

A film featuring three young men who discuss the difficulties of becoming fathers at an early age. Available from New Dimension Films, 85895 Lorane Highway, Eugene, OR 97405, (503) 484-7125.

* For Church Settings.

APPENDIX G
AIDS RESOURCES FOR THE CLASSROOM

AIDS: A Risky Business for Everyone

Intended as a supplement to the *Sex Respect* curriculum. Comes in three separate workbooks: one for teachers, one for students, one for parents. Contains the medical facts, refutes safe sex, and teaches prevention. Available from Respect, Inc., P.O. Box 349, Bradley, IL 60915, (815) 932-8389.

AIDS and the Education of Our Children: Guide for Parents and Teachers

A booklet for parents and teachers. Covers the medical facts and how to protect young people. Available from the U. S. Department of Education, 400 Maryland Ave. SW, Room 4019, Washington, DC 20202, (202) 732-4024.

AIDS and Young People

A booklet for use in public school classrooms. Presents the medical facts and how to avoid getting AIDS. Available from two sources: Concerned Women for America, 370 L'Enfant Promenade SW, Suite 800, Washington, DC 20024, (800) 458-8797, and Project Respect, Committee on the Status of Women, Box 97, Golf, IL 60029, (312) 729-3298.

AIDS—Learn and Live

A video for seventh through twelfth grade public school students. Interviews with physicians, teens, and AIDS victims. Shows how to say no. Available from Teen-Aid, N. 1330 Calispel, Spokane, WA 99201, (509) 466-8679.

AIDS: Learn for Your Life

A film which encourages sexual abstinence to reduce the risk of disease. New Dimension Films, 85895 Lorane Highway, Eugene, OR 97405, (503) 484-7125.

Living Safely in the Age of AIDS

A 10-lesson curriculum for classroom usage. Each lesson includes description, review questions, and discussion questions. For more information, contact: National AIDS Prevention Institute, P.O. Box 2500, Culpeper, VA 22701, (703) 825-4040.

Who Do You Listen To?: Sex in the Age of AIDS

A film intended for public secondary schools. Covers the medical facts and how to make the right decisions. Check about free lending policy to public schools. Available from Gospel Films, Box 455, Muskegon, MI 49443, (800) 253-0413.

Will 'Safe Sex' Education Effectively Combat AIDS?

An informal paper that abstracts research showing the fallacy of safe sex. An excellent reference available from the U. S. Department of Education, 400 Maryland Ave. S.W., Room 4019, Washington, DC 20202, (202) 732-4024.

APPENDIX H
PAMPHLETS FOR TEENS

Best Birth Control for Teens. Womanity, 1700 Oak Park Blvd., Room C-4, Pleasant Hill, CA 94523, (415) 943-6424.

Chastity Is Sexual Goodness. Womanity (see above).

Dating Decisions I Can Live With. Teen-Aid, N. 1330 Calispel, Spokane, WA 99201, (509) 466-8679.

Dating Guide for Guys 'n Girls. Womanity (see above).

First Aid for AIDS. Womanity (see above).

Gone All the Way—Now Where? Womanity (see above).

Health and Sexual Ethics. Womanity (see above).

How to Say No. Womanity (see above).

I'm Saving Myself for Brooke Shields. Pamphlets, Box 424, Burlington, IA 52601.

Is There Real Safe Sex? Teen-Aid (see above).

Knowing Is Caring and Caring Is Sharing. Life Cycle Books, P.O. Box 792, Lewiston, NY 14092-0792, (416) 690-5860.

Many Teens Are Saying 'No.' U. S. Department of HHS, Government Printing Office, Washington, DC 20402.

No Is a Love Word. Human Life Center, University of Steubenville, Steubenville, OH 43952, (614) 282-9953.

No—the Positive Answer. Why Wait?, Josh McDowell Ministries, Box 1000, Dallas, TX 95221, (214) 907-1000.

On the Verge of Virginity. Womanity (see above).

Saying No, the Way to Grow. Life Cycle Books (see above).

Secondary Virginity. Womanity (see above).

Sex Outside Marriage. Womanity (see above).

Sexual Common Sense: Affirming Adolescent Abstinence. Womanity (see above).

Teen Esteem. Womanity (see above).

Understanding Sexuality. Focus on the Family, Pomona, CA 91799, (714) 620-8500.

Virginity, Beautiful and Free. Womanity (see above).

Wait. Project Respect, Box 97, Golf, IL 60029.

Why Chastity? Couple to Couple League, Box 11084, Cincinnati, OH 45211, (513) 661-7612.

You're the One. Teen-Aid (see above).

APPENDIX I
LIST OF TABLES

I. FAMILY PLANNING PROGRAMS FOR ADOLESCENTS

1. Significant Events in the History of Contemporary Family Planning
2. Federal Programs Through the U.S. Department of HHS That Address the Problem of Adolescent Pregnancy (1986)
3. Federal Expenditures on Family Planning; Births and Abortions to Women 15-19; Pregnancies, Births, and Abortions per 1,000 Women 15-19, 1970-1981.
4. Impact of Teenage Family Planning Programs.
5. Adolescent Pregnancy Rates and Outcomes, 1970-1982.
6. Rates of Teenage Pregnancy and Abortion, plus Unmarried Births for States with FNCC.
7. Number of Teens/% of Female Teenagers Served 1970-1975.
8. Physicians' Comparison of Contraceptive Availability With Level of Teenage Sexual Activity.

II. SCHOOL-BASED CLINICS FOR ADOLESCENTS

9. SBCs and Contraceptives

III. COMPREHENSIVE SEX EDUCATION

10. 24 States Have Mandatory AIDS Education in Schools
11. 8 States Have a Mandatory AIDS Curriculum
12. At What Level Is AIDS Education Introduced?
13. Piaget's Stages of Cognitive Development
14. Concrete vs Formal Operator
15. Cognitive Development and Decisions About Sexual Activity
16. Cognitive Development as It Pertains to Love
17. Kohlberg's Stages of Moral Reasoning

IV. INFLUENCING TODAY'S YOUTH

18. Estimated Shifts in the Influences Upon 13- to 19-year-olds Who Change Their Values and Behavior
19. Trends in Conception Among Women 15-19 Years of Age
20. Percentage of Never-Married Teenagers Having Had Sexual Intercourse, Based on Parental Strictness, 1983
21. Percentage of Never-Married Teenagers Having Had Sexual Intercourse, Based on Number of Parental Dating Rules, 1983
22. Percentage of Teenage Girls Having Sexual Intercourse, Based on the Age Dating Began

V. ABSTINENCE EDUCATION

23. Items Teenagers Consider to Be a Problem
24-28. Effectiveness of the Project Respect Program
29. Impact of Abstinence Program on Teen Pregnancies and Grades
30. Effectiveness of the Teen Choice Program

VI. PARENTAL INVOLVEMENT

31. Attitudes of Young People About Sex and Sexuality
32. Attitudes of Parents About Sex and Sexuality
33. Teenage Pregnancy Rate